A Life in Trauma

Dr Chris Luke qualified in 1982 at University College Dublin and has been an emergency physician for over 35 years. He has worked in frontline medicine in Ireland, the UK and Australia, and has been a consultant in emergency medicine in Cork for over 20 years. Luke, who calls himself a 'slightly militant altruist', is a passionate and outspoken advocate for the public health service, those who depend on it and those who work in it. He has four children and lives in Cork.

A Life in Trauma

Memoirs of an Emergency Physician

Dr Chris Luke

Gill Books

Gill Books
Hume Avenue
Park West
Dublin 12
www.gillbooks.ie

Gill Books is an imprint of M.H. Gill and Co.

978 07171 9141 3

Designed by Síofra Murphy
Edited by Sheila Armstrong
Proofread by Caroline Twomey

Printed by Sprintprint, Dublin
This book is typeset in Adobe Caslon.

A CIP catalogue record for this book is available from the British Library.

5

For Victoria
You (still) bring me joy!

Trauma

(1) n. a deeply distressing or disturbing experience;
(2) n. physical injury.

Contents

Author's Note on Emergency Medicine

Emergency Medicine is a legally recognised speciality of medical practice in Ireland, focused on providing immediate, urgently required care. It is practised mainly in hospital emergency departments (EDs); historically (and still in the UK) these units were known as casualty and then accident and emergency (A&E) departments, but the re-naming in Ireland 20 years ago was designed to make the purpose and function of the unit as unambiguous as possible. The speciality is one of the largest and fastest growing disciplines in the English-speaking world, although it remains relatively under-resourced in Ireland in terms of facilities and staffing.

There are about 28 public and six private EDs in the country. The public departments are open to all-comers 'in a crisis' 24 hours a day, every day, but they've been oversubscribed for decades and are often overcrowded. The main reasons for this – among many – are that there are too few hospital beds or step-down facilities to admit patients for long-term care; the departments themselves are often poorly designed and too small (even the ones that were opened recently); and the EDs are often perceived as the only available portal into hospital care for those on long waiting lists or those with particularly complex needs. Notwithstanding these challenges, emergency medicine has a very proud tradition of providing urgent, effective care for around a quarter of the population of the Anglophone world, as well as offering profoundly important leadership and innovation across great swathes of healthcare. I believe that Irish EDs are beacons of hope and care in a sometimes-frightening world, but they are also locations of human and organisational imperfection.

Prologue

'The past is never dead. It's not even past.'
(William Faulkner)

I've always thought that the old schoolyard phrase 'sticks and stones may break my bones, but names will never hurt me' couldn't really be true. Because every teenager knows that words can wound, and every politician knows that a powerful speech can trigger warfare or bring about a ceasefire. Sadly, in my own case, mere words spelled near disaster for my career as an emergency physician. In hindsight, I suppose it was apt that it took an actual tragedy to trigger my calamitous outburst.

On 10 February 2011, a 19-seater Manx2 commuter plane left Belfast at about 8.10 a.m. – a little late, but less than 40 minutes later the twin turboprop was approaching Cork airport. Unfortunately, dense fog cloaked the airport so completely that its landing lights and markings were invisible from the terminal and the flight deck of the plane, several hundred feet up in the air. Air traffic controllers instructed the pilots to circle rather than attempt landing blind, and, for the next hour, the plane did just that while safer landing conditions were sought in Kerry, Shannon and Waterford.

But the efforts to find an alternative place to land proved futile and, at about 9.46 a.m., the Cork tower instructed the aircraft to begin its descent. As the plane neared the western Runway 17, it rolled suddenly to the left, and then to the right. Its wingtip touched the ground at speed and the plane flipped over onto its roof, veering violently to the right and then ploughing through the grass beside the landing strip. At roughly 9.50 a.m., it came to a standstill, its nose buried in soil 70 metres from the centre of the runway, and both engines caught fire.

Four miles away, in the centre of Cork, I was sitting on stage in the packed ballroom of the Metropole Hotel, about to go live on air on Pat Kenny's RTÉ morning radio show. I had been invited to talk about the 'trolley crisis' in Cork's emergency departments – an issue I thought exceptionally important and in need of urgent public discussion. But I was already hoping I could get away quickly, anxious about spending too long away from the busy emergency department in the nearby Mercy Hospital, where I was due to work that morning.

As I sat there, listening to the other guests, I couldn't help recalling the words of an old school friend, the son of an eminent paediatrician, who'd once chided me about ventilating on the subject of healthcare: 'Jeez, Chris, you medics are always moaning. You just can't help yourselves.'

Still, I was determined to have my say that morning. After countless cruel months, I was at my wit's end with the conditions in the two departments in which I was then working, and definitely not in the mood to offer a positive spin on things. The truth was that the atmosphere in both units had turned into a noxious fug of anguish, despair and hostility, with patients on trolleys as far as the eye could see, and many more hidden in nooks, crannies, back corridors or side rooms. Standing by most trolleys, there were usually partners or adult children proactively representing the interests of the often-elderly occupants. It was like getting through a thronged obstacle course whenever a call went out for staff to hurry to Resuscitation ('Resus'), or to one of the cubicles for a cardiac arrest, a newly arrived road accident victim or an overdose case. And, every day, ambulances queued outside to offload their urgent cargo, while dozens of the 'walking wounded' sat or stood for hours in the reception area, as they waited for their name to be called by the Triage nurse.

By 2011, I'd endured such conditions for over twenty years, and it was obvious that things were getting steadily worse. Shortages of space, staff and alternatives to the hospital emergency department meant that the joke that 'A&E' stood for 'Anything & Everything' was no longer funny. It had become the default position. And the results were not just deeply unpleasant conditions for the sick and their carers – they were genuinely toxic.

Some of my medical colleagues had calculated that dozens of people were dying every year in Ireland's crowded emergency departments (EDs) because the urgency of their conditions was not recognised amid the mayhem. Self-evidently, our patients could not receive the sort of humane, effective and well-organised care of which we all dreamed, and for which we had trained for so long and so hard. And the most alarming consequence for me was that experienced nursing staff were leaving in droves, while those that stayed seldom smiled. In truth, then, I was well beyond exasperated. I was actually seething with an anger that was completely at odds with the light-hearted atmosphere of the radio show.

Inside the crushed aircraft, the two pilots and four passengers at the front had been killed instantly by a combination of head, chest and abdominal injuries. Six other occupants towards the rear were trapped in their seats, in total darkness, as the lights went out on impact. One of them, a regular commuter between Cork and Belfast, subsequently recounted how the crumpled fuselage was pressing upon his head, and he felt he was being suffocated as mud and water poured into the cabin.

He could also hear the screams of a woman nearby, who later remembered that in the first few seconds post-impact, she held her neighbour's hand and they prayed together, terrified that they'd survived the crash only to be incinerated by the flames discernible through the windows on both sides. Moments later, there was a banging on the sides of the plane and its windows, and cries of 'Don't panic! We're going to get you out!' from the airport rescue teams. The survivors weren't long receiving assistance. A fleet of eight ambulances was already on its way, along with numerous fire, rescue and airport police vehicles, bearing about two hundred personnel to the crash site. And, soon after, a tent was hastily erected near the scene of devastation to serve as a temporary morgue while, inside the downed aircraft, the grim task of medical assessment of the victims, living and dead, got underway.

Conscious that I was under pressure to get back to work, Pat had invited me up on the Metropole stage so we could chat briefly before the main interviews – with two of Cork's leading politicians, Micheál Martin and Simon Coveney – of the morning. As he did so, Pat mentioned that there were 'reports coming in' of some sort of incident at the airport. I was immediately on edge, as I knew I would be routinely involved in any 'major incident' response. Then Pat said, 'Chris Luke, would you very quickly give us your thoughts on the situation in the emergency department in CUH, which we've heard so much about this week? And I mean – *other* than the shortages of beds?'

He was probably referring to a piece in the *Irish Examiner* a few days before that was headed, 'Hospital's A&E "swamped" by 4,411 patients'. The report described how the number of patients attending the emergency department at Cork University Hospital (CUH) had reached 142 a day, with a 'shocking trolley count' and 'higher than usual' waiting times. The Health Service Executive (HSE) had confirmed that the figures were accurate and unprecedented, but not entirely the HSE's fault. They pointed out that 58 per cent of the people attending the department were not admitted to a hospital bed, and this contributed to the ED overcrowding, as did the frailty and advanced age of many patients, and the need to isolate suspected cases of Swine Flu in some wards, making their beds unavailable for other patients.

What the paper hadn't reported was the endless despairing email correspondence between myself and the other consultants in the department at CUH about the seemingly permanent chaos within, the wretchedness of everyone on and around the dozens of trolleys, and the impossibility of finding a space to examine even the most urgent patients with a modicum of privacy.

Worst of all were the countless 'near-misses', or people whose life-threatening medical conditions the more experienced senior staff kept spotting in the packed waiting room, or on chairs in dark corners. It went without saying that our capacity to address patients' pain, fear and indignity was severely compromised. It was now so bad that the department there was sometimes described as being like the 'Black Hole of Calcutta'.

Bad as this description was, the real problem for me was that the Irish media had been full of stories about the terrible 'emergency levels on A&E trolleys' exactly twelve months before. And, five years previously, then Minister for Health Mary Harney had said that the overcrowding of the state's emergency departments needed to be treated as a 'national emergency'. Indeed, over the previous 15 years, I had repeatedly made the front pages of the local *Echo*, not just in Cork, but in Liverpool too, pleading for help with the intolerable overcrowding.

So it was a case of severe déjà vu, in January and February 2011, to see the local press in Cork full of articles about the intractable overcrowding in the city's two EDs. The only difference on this occasion was that I finally snapped. Boiling over with a rage I'd bottled up for 25 years, I answered Pat Kenny's question as to what was 'causing' the endless crisis in the country's emergency departments, *beyond* the bed shortage. And I was extraordinarily blunt.

I said that the problem was about *far more* than bed numbers, and that literally *everyone* had a part to play in its causation and resolution. Like the CEOs of our public hospitals, who were so seldom seen 'leading' in their emergency departments, in contrast with the situation in the NHS in England, where senior administrators were subject to severe sanctions if the overall patients' waiting time in their hospital's A&E department exceeded just four hours.

Like the handful of GPs who kept referring non-emergency cases to the *emergency* department. I cited a case I'd seen just the day before, in CUH, when a patient with a two-year history of a sore shoulder was referred by his GP to the ED despite the protests of the patient's family. He and they had waited hours before being told – predictably – that they needed to see a shoulder specialist, and an outpatient clinic referral letter would have to be written for him. The reason? Clear instructions had been issued by the surgeons that they would not see long-term cases referred through the 'back door' of the ED.

That morning, in answer to Pat Kenny's question, I also observed that there seemed, in theory at least, to be a risk of what health economists call 'a perverse incentive', whereby a GP got paid even if he or she referred every second patient to the local ED – which didn't receive a fee for referred patients, regardless of the extent of tests or treatment undertaken.

For good measure, I added that attention also needed to be paid to the 'productivity' of some young doctors in our EDs, or at least that of the *locums* who so often staffed them but sometimes seemed to undertake a pitiful amount of work during a typical shift.

I contrasted this with the workload of junior doctors 'in my day' (what else can an older doctor say?), when a first- or second-year graduate might be expected to see and sort a dozen or more cases over eight hours. Worse still, I used a description of first-year doctors that my medical peers and

I regularly employed in reminiscences about our own early medical days: 'When I was a baby doctor ...'

In retrospect, I was caught off-guard by Pat's leading questions (he hinted a little mischievously at widespread laziness among young medics, which I certainly wasn't diagnosing), and in the intense heat of the moment, stressed by the rumour of a major incident in progress and the decades-old difficulties of ED overcrowding, my language was more muddled and emotive than my usual thoughtful utterances. My second mistake was in echoing his tone. 'Well, you might say that, Pat, but I couldn't possibly comment.' (Laughter around the room.)

Still, tongue-tied or not, I was as polite as I could manage about a situation where some of my patients were actually dying and countless more were suffering – *avoidably* – and a terrible injustice seemed to be involved. And then, glancing at my phone, I read the text message: 'Major Incident Declared. Contact CUH.' I stood up and quickly made my excuses, leaving the two political big-hitters arguing over what I had said – or *meant* to say.

When it comes to a major incident, or disaster, there are two fundamental initial measures required of a major trauma centre like CUH. The first is to send out a trained medical team to attend the incident site.

The second is to empty the hospital's ED, as far as possible, to make space for the incoming casualties, and to marshal a team of two or three staff to manage each victim as they arrive, in the best available area. The ideal space is Resus but, in practice, other rooms and cubicles are usually used too.

My job when I got to CUH that morning, ten minutes or so after leaving the Metropole, was to help clear the department by moving patients up to other wards or, better still, discharging them. Pushing the interview to the back of my mind, I undertook a rapid round of our inpatient ward, the clinical decision unit (CDU), where patients with potentially severe illness or injury are admitted under our care until their suspected conditions 'crystallise or dematerialise'.

I was blessed that morning, because Anna Dillon, one of those wonderful nurses who combines vast experience with practical solutions and a calming smile, was in charge, and we were able to allow most of the patients to go home, just as the first survivors of the Manx2 crash began to arrive in the CDU after their assessment in Resus. And once the situation was becoming clear, the limited number of survivors was confirmed and their conditions stabilised, I was able to get a lift in a Garda car down to the Mercy, where I was actually scheduled to work.

Cork's inner-city ED at the Mercy had one of its busiest ever days that day, as patients were diverted there from its sister hospital. Still, we coped as always with the surge in caseload. And, of course, all the other usual work continued too, in the city-centre ED and at CUH, where numbers quickly climbed back to their supersaturated normal by midnight. That evening, it was clear from telephone conversations with colleagues at CUH that the overall emergency response was thought to have gone reasonably well.

The airport crash that morning led to an appalling loss of life, and I couldn't stop thinking about the poor relatives of those who had died that day. But at least the frequently rehearsed emergency response at Cork airport had been reasonably efficient. We had helped those who could be helped, we had learned important lessons for the next time and we had survived another gruelling day in the health service trenches.

The following morning, the sky fell in on my head.

I'd had little chance to reflect on my performance on the *Pat Kenny Show*, but the then President of the Irish Medical Organisation (IMO), Professor Sean Tierney, emailed me to say that there had been an 'unprecedented number' of calls and emails to IMO offices the previous day from GPs and non-consultant doctors who were 'shocked and upset' by my comments. Younger colleagues at CUH urged me not to go on Twitter, because the hostility towards me online was 'incredible' and had gone viral. And the Irish College of General Practitioners and numerous local GPs had apparently contacted the CEO of CUH to request my suspension or, at the very least, 'disciplining'. And it got steadily worse.

Over the following hours, days and weeks, I was blanked or ignored by dozens of doctors-in-training in hospital corridors and on the city's streets, and I received abusive phone calls, letters and messages from GPs everywhere. The backlash created increasing difficulty for me in my professional and personal life, but the ostracism was easily the most painful and disabling aspect of the whole affair. In my nearly 30 years of practice, I had never felt so alone – or isolated – within the profession. In truth, even if it wasn't obvious to anyone other than my wife, I was shattered by the tsunami of animosity, the cold-shouldering, and the blighted reputation. And I was shaken by the subsequent disciplinary process in the CEO's office at CUH, despite the support of

Cork's leading employment lawyer. Indeed, my mental health and professional confidence were so damaged by the effort to 'cancel' me online, in the medical press, and in person, that I was obliged to take several weeks' leave in April 2011.

It was an ignominious fall from grace for a medic whom the Minister for Health had described the year before as 'one of the leading emergency medical physicians in the country', and who had built a career on being – above all – likeable, enthusiastic and kind. It was also a bizarre sort of calamity: it wasn't as if I was fabricating or exaggerating the facts. If anything, I'd been relatively restrained in my examples of the unspoken causes of the bedlam in our EDs. But my choice of *words* – in which I am normally so careful – was truly disastrous for my once-promising career. Looking back almost in disbelief at that fateful morning, I remember feeling as if I had recklessly steered my own vessel onto the rocks. Now the only important question was: could it be salvaged?

The Letter

It is a truth almost universally acknowledged nowadays that distressing adversity or psychological trauma at an early age can have a damaging and enduring effect on some individuals, even when the adverse experience may seem to others to be minor, or barely worth mentioning. For reasons that were once intensely private, I agree. This is because I still clearly recall one particularly traumatic moment in my own childhood, the impact of which has reverberated through my personal and professional life, for decades. And yet, looking back now, it must sound remarkably trivial to some.

It was on a wintry weekday evening in late 1970, I think, when my mother and I had our unforeseen moment of painful revelation. I was eleven years old at the time, a rather lonely, only child, routinely left to his own devices at home. Home was a semi-detached bungalow in Stillorgan, built in the 1950s at what was then the edge of Dublin, but gloomily decorated in a sort of Edwardian pastiche style by my middle-aged mother. At that time, she was working in the Guinness Press Office in St James' Gate, in the city centre, a good hour's drive through the evening rush-hour traffic, and I generally got back from school in Ballsbridge a couple of hours before her. In those days, I'd try to get my homework done quickly before trawling around, eternally bored, looking for something to do or to read. TV was only an occasional treat, when my mother rented one of those machines with a coin slot at the side, a long-forgotten feature of the olden days. And the radio held little appeal for a schoolboy. The boys on the road had all gone in, and our Siamese cat, Ming, was a haughty and unsympathetic companion.

So mostly it was a choice between re-reading our 1920s version of the *Children's Encyclopaedia*, with its Aesop's Fables, sepia pictures of Egyptian pyramids, famous ships like the *Lusitania* and *Titanic*, and monstrous Amazonian anacondas, or working my way through the extensive collection of hardcover books and paperbacks by Ngaio Marsh, Mary Renault or Antonia Fraser and the like. But by 1970, I'd truly exhausted most of the material that suited even the most precocious of children. I don't know what prompted me to open the two-drawer filing cabinet that stood in the hall, under an antimacassar, one of those small bits of cloth draped over furniture in Victorian times. Idle curiosity, I suppose. Or what made me root through umpteen dusty files within, mostly relating to income tax, credit unions or Arthur Guinness Son & Co. (Dublin) Ltd. But my inquisitiveness and boredom yielded a letter that swiftly and frighteningly perplexed me.

The typed letter was addressed to the proprietor of a hotel in County Donegal, in 1961 or thereabouts, and it seemed to be from my late father, Leslie Luke. At least, that was the name at the bottom of the page. But in the letter, *this* Leslie Luke was writing to the hotelier to confirm that he would be arriving the following week with his *wife, Doreen*, and numerous children. That was what completely stumped me. Nothing in this seemingly straightforward missive made any sense. My father had died tragically in 1963, after an operation, I knew, but I was his only son, surely? And the only Doreen I'd ever heard of was my Aunty Doreen, a kindly friend of my mother's who used to take me for birthday treats to places like the Royal Marine or Fullers Café in Dún Laoghaire, and who gave me presents like wallets, handkerchiefs and books. So who was this other Doreen, and how did the children fit into the puzzle?

I sat on the hall floor clutching the letter, baffled. No obvious solutions presented themselves to me, but there was a gnawing sensation in my stomach, and a profound submerged anxiety was returning, the one from a long time before. The house was silent. Dusk had settled in by then, and the only light in the hallway was from a tiny red lantern containing a diminutive Christ, above my mother's bedroom door. Reflexively, I moved into her room and sat on the end of the bed, without turning on the light. Therefore, it was to a completely darkened house that my mother got home, an hour or so later. I could hear the concern in her voice as she unlocked the front door and called out, 'Christopher? Where are you?'

In response, I mumbled, 'In here.'

She came in and switched on the light in her room.

'What's going on?' she asked, frowning.

'Mum, what's this?' I replied, handing her the letter I'd been clutching for well over an hour.

I recall to this day the colour draining from her face as she recognised and re-read the letter she had herself probably typed for Leslie Luke, my father and her boss. I remember her sitting down beside me and trembling as she mumbled her answers.

This moment of crisis remains indelibly etched in my memory, even though the precise words she uttered were suddenly of no consequence and all that mattered to me was the Truth.

'Mum, are you actually my mother?' I asked, dreading the answer.

'Yes, Christopher. I am. I really am. But, you see, your father and I weren't married. He was married to Doreen…'

'You mean, Aunty Doreen?'

'Yes. Her name is Doreen Luke.'

'But what about all the children?'

'Your dad had six other children.'

'Was he really my father?'

'Yes.'

'And are you really, truly my mother?'

'Yes.'

'Honest?'

'Honestly, I am. Please believe me. I am your mother.'

Shaking with fear, I got up, retreated to my own bedroom, and got under the covers. And I prayed, fervently, that God would keep my mother alive for as long as He could, so that I could stay, and not have to leave again.

My whispered prayers were both heartfelt and eloquent because, even by the age of eleven, I was well-versed in the contents of an Irish Roman Catholic missal, and capable of reciting a range of prayers for hours at a time, to God, the

Blessed Virgin Mary and my Guardian Angel, especially. In fact, while Dubliners often say for effect, 'I had it beaten into me', I suspect I really did. Because I had been initially educated as a proper sinner, the very product of sin indeed, in an orphanage.

St Philomena's Orphanage was situated in the former mansion of the Pilkington family, Westbury, at the top of the Upper Kilmacud Road in Stillorgan, in South County Dublin. It had also been run as a residential institution for boys and girls ('the children of unmarried mothers') since 1932 by the Daughters of Charity of St Vincent de Paul. And then, in the mid-1960s, the Archbishop of Dublin, John Charles McQuaid, arranged for the convent and its grounds to be converted into a secondary school for girls, to be called Marillac. God only knows how many real orphans it had once contained. Legend, which remains the quintessential feature of my early years, has it that I was handed to a local woman in Kilmacud when I was two weeks of age, and then to the originally French order of nuns by my mother when I was six months old, 'because they weren't as harsh as the Irish orders', and that I spent most of the next six years living in St Philomena's. But the truth is that I simply don't know. I've never had more than faint memories of the period, and I've spent most of my life trying not to bring them to the surface more than necessary.

I do vaguely recall bunk-beds, with cold metal bars and thin pillows. And prayers in dark dormitories. Statues of Mary in abundance, and Mass in a little convent chapel. The high infants' classroom. The hairy legs of a young nun sitting on a table reading to a gaggle of small children, while I snuck under the table. The big fields and farm at the back of the convent, with herds of brown cattle and a mesmerizingly busy dairy. Jim, the farmer, who would sometimes take me on tractor rides around the ploughed fields. Cow parsley, cowpats and dung beetles. Giant trees lining the long drive and narrow lanes within the demesne. A huge kitchen with young women bustling about. Clotted white sauce swamping bacon, bitter greens and watery mashed potato. Luminous ornamental flowerbeds in front of the big house. Shiny parquet floors and a grandfather clock ticking loudly in the convent's front parlour, where I would sit quietly towards the end, with my mother and one or more elderly nuns, at a huge, gleaming mahogany table that gave off an intense waxy fragrance. The smell of fear.

There were times when I got out of the orphanage. To Sunshine Homes around Dublin county, to the amateur home cinema run for the orphanage children by kindly locals in the old Baumann's complex in Stillorgan and, periodically – like a few other lucky children – to an actual home. In my case, this was at No. 33, Oaktree Road in Stillorgan, a few hundred yards from St Philomena's, which my mother had purchased in 1961. And once, at least, I believe I was even taken away by my parents for a flying visit to Wales. But to a little fellow, there must have been an eternity between these outings, which in hindsight were meticulously orchestrated. Indeed, it's clear in retrospect that the charming black-and-white snaps of my father, mother and me, with Billy the cat, were carefully shot by one of Dublin's top photographers in the 1960s, Tony O'Malley, who was regularly hired by my father and mother for their Guinness PR work. So there were carefully crafted 'happy memories' on film, which now seem strangely sweet, but fake.

It turns out, too, that a great deal of planning had gone into my eventual release from St Philomena's. At some stage, when I was about six or seven, I understand, I was extricated from the orphanage, which was being wound down in advance of the building of the new Marillac school, and I moved to No. 33 to live with my mother. Or rather my 'aunt', as she initially described herself to the neighbours, in explaining the sudden arrival of her 'poor nephew', even if his piercing brown eyes and Roman nose bore an uncanny resemblance to her own. Cleary the veil was flimsy, and my story raised more than a few eyebrows.

It is striking, though, that once I had moved to Oaktree Road, my new life became vividly memorable, even if my identity was uncertain and the locals didn't quite know what to call me. So, from the age of six or seven, I remember an old Morris Minor in the driveway, later replaced by a Mini. A tricycle, too. And after Billy, an ancient grey tomcat, a series of Siamese cats, Ming and Ching.

Of course, living on a suburban estate, away from the previous confinement, there were suddenly lots of other new children, laughing, leaping and running around. There were friendly mothers chatting at doorsteps. Serious dads heading off to work in the morning, in their cars, or on foot to the bus stop. There were front gardens to play in, often in non-ornamental flowerbeds that could be turned into battlefields or building sites. And back gardens with clotheslines and tiny orchards of two or three apple and pear trees. And the field just a hundred yards away, for playing football and hide-and-seek in the adjacent woods. There was the gang of boys from nearby houses: John and Stephen Conway from No. 50, just opposite No. 33, David Delahunt,

Eugene ('Nudge') Harrington and James Dormer from homes on both sides of the Conways, and the effervescent Gannons next-door in No. 35.

What fun we had. And what blissful freedom. Beyond the houses and the field to the south lay Brewery Road and, behind a low boundary wall, was the river that ran along its edge, from the Leopardstown Inn through the Esso administration grounds, until it passed under the Brewery ruins and the Stillorgan Road and on into the grounds of St John of God's Hospital. And in the opposite direction was the old Harcourt Street to Leopardstown railway line, closed in 1958, which provided a magnificently leafy, linear playground for all the children of the area. And play we did, for endless hours it seemed, until all the light had gone from the day. Football, kerbies, scutting, doorbells. Boyish mischief galore, like the time we pushed a banger through a letterbox one October evening, and ran for our dear lives when the curtain unexpectedly caught fire. Understandably, the enraged house owner, Mr McNulty, drove around the estate at breakneck speed until he'd rounded up all six of us, and drove us straight down to the car park of Blackrock Garda Station. Here, in return for not being presented to the duty desk sergeant, we readily agreed to go to our respective homes and confess to our parents what had happened. Now that was memorable, as was the smack or two of the wooden spoon that my mother wielded that evening (for the medical record, I was merely an accomplice!).

There were also the Saturday matinees in the Ormonde cinema in Stillorgan (the wonderfully bloody *Ambush Bay*, circa 1967, comes instantly to mind, and the perennials, *Laurel and Hardy*), the 'Cubs' in Glenalbyn, and the odd accident or crisis. I recall wandering off one afternoon and finding myself in the front room of a boy I'd met once before en route to the railway line to pick blackberries. Realising that we'd been playing with his Subbuteo football game for a rather long time, and that it was now dark, I thanked the mother of the house politely and wandered back down Leopardstown Road towards home, only to be met by search parties from my own road who'd been out looking for me for hours. Such was the care-free, or *care-less*, life of an ex-orphanage boy, as he engaged slowly at first, but then with relish, with the boys and girls and mothers and fathers of Oaktree Road and its environs.

There were occasional uncomfortable reminders of St Philomena's. Like the dreary processions on Holy Days, winding their way around the roads of the Merville Estate, decked with white and gold papal flags and bunting, to the old St Lawrence's Church in Kilmacud, where the legendary parish priest, Father Harley, would celebrate endless Mass, a half-mile from the front gates of the former orphanage. And then there were oddly comforting hymns, like 'Soul of My Saviour' or 'Tantum Ergo', classics of the late 1960s. In fact, the most disturbing reminder was provided by the formidable women in the playground on Library Road, in Dún Laoghaire, where my mother would deposit me on a Saturday while she selected her half-dozen books to borrow in the Carnegie Library across the road. I recall my regular slight panic when, at 3.00 p.m., they would suddenly lock the gates and herd all the children into the adjacent hall for obligatory prayers. No one was allowed out until these were concluded. (I learned latterly that one of the shepherdesses was a Dominican nun, in civvies.)

There were many benign neighbours, thankfully, like the kindly Mr Dunne, a few houses up, who I recognised from the local church or orphanage cinema outings. And there were the nameless, impassive women in houses in the Merville Estate and Montrose who minded me perfunctorily for a few hours at a time, while my mother went to work. And a countrywoman from Wexford who arrived at No. 33 every so often, when I was seven or eight, to take me for bus trips to Shankill beach, a stone's throw from Loughlinstown Hospital, and whose specialty was white bread and sugar sandwiches. My mother was not best pleased when she later learned about this diet, but Mr Cotter, the dentist in Donnybrook, who had to repair the damage, must have been delighted.

My maternal grandparents featured prominently in my mother's conversations on the phone, but I recall only a few visits to their redbrick terraced house in Beechwood Avenue in Ranelagh, with its authentically Edwardian decoration and furniture. The house was only a few doors away from 'where Maureen O'Hara and Jack MacGowran used to play' with my mother in the 1920s and 1930s, she'd say, although those legendary actors' names meant little to me. My mother made it plain that she thought my grandmother, Christina (or Pidge, as she was known) was a 'very difficult' woman, who had for years needed a great deal of nursing at home by her only daughter.

Mostly confined to a chair or bed because of her varicose veins, her thyroid disease and her weight, she tended to glower at me and her daughter, while my grandfather, Christopher, or Christy, Redmond, impeccably dressed in a three-piece suit with a fob watch, always seemed to be preoccupied with lighting fires or lighting his pipe. He said very little, I recall, and I used to get the feeling that he too was secretly keen to avoid his spouse's glare. While she was largely unforthcoming on the subject of Pidge, my mother was forever devoted to her dad. The second eldest of eight siblings from Lennox Street, near the South Circular Road, Christy had had an energetic early existence: as a young man, he was said to have regularly cycled from the city centre in Dublin to Wicklow, and he was an avid supporter of Shamrock Rovers.

But he reserved most of his youthful zeal for politics, it seems, becoming an enthusiastic supporter of Home Rule within John Redmond's Irish Parliamentary Party. Initially described as a 'stenographer' (in the 1911 Census), he later served as a private parliamentary secretary to the populist 'Wee Joe' Devlin, the *Irish News* journalist and Catholic nationalist MP for West Belfast, and later Tyrone, which meant that he spent much of his time rotating between Dublin, Westminster and Belfast, which was seemingly a source of exasperation for his wife. In a subsequent career, prompted by the shattering effect of the 1916 Rising and the 1918 Conscription Crisis on Redmondite nationalism and 'Home Rule incrementalism' (followed by the sudden death of John Redmond, in March 1918), my grandfather became a senior reporter and music critic at the *Irish Times*. And it was in that capacity, I subsequently learned, that he first met and mentored one Leslie Luke, who was starting out as a journalist.

The only other maternal relative that I ever met as a little boy was my uncle, Garry Redmond. Later the editor of the *RTÉ Guide*, he was a brilliant Synge Street-educated, legally trained author and sports journalist with the *Irish Independent*, *Irish Press* and *Observer*, who liked to spar verbally with my mother, his older only sibling. Every time I saw them together, they embarked on a perennial game of interrupting each other's interruptions. My mother would regularly tell me that her baby brother had broken her favourite toy doll when he was a toddler, and she seemed never to have forgiven him. She also resented the fact that she'd had to walk him to school in Rathmines every morning for years and so was unable to mix with other girls her own age. But most of all, there seemed to be a never-ending rivalry between the siblings to be the most interesting conversationalist at any gathering. The reality was that one was as good – and as garrulous – as the other.

I always enjoyed my visits to see Garry, who lived, in the late 1960s, with his elegant and good-natured wife, Annette, in a splendid apartment on Raglan Road, near my school in Ballsbridge. His erudite, rugby-focused banter was a balm to my little ears. Sadly, even at that stage, I always felt that he and his sister tolerated each other but not much more, so I only got to meet him once or twice a year, particularly after he and Annette moved to Dalkey.

Much as I enjoyed the occasional after-school visits to the Redmonds, my favourite hosts were the wives of my mother's work team. I had no idea then that this is what they were, but in the latter years of the 1960s a sort of network of these (and a couple of other) women took it upon themselves to support my unmarried mother by minding her son. Regardless of their own inclinations, I realise now that this made some sense as their husbands were involved in an increasingly successful enterprise, producing the quarterly *Harp* magazine, the house journal of Arthur Guinness & Son, then one of the largest, wealthiest and most benign employers in Dublin.

My father had been the Press Officer for Guinness, and Editor of the *Harp*, which had evolved from being a rather content-light newsletter for employees, first published in 1958, to a serious and eventually glossy house journal for which the staff paid a nominal sum, and impressive contributors were relatively well remunerated in those straitened times. My mother was the Editorial Secretary, as well as his 'other woman', and when Leslie died suddenly, following abdominal surgery in Monkstown Hospital in August 1963, she had taken over the reins of the magazine, which had gone from strength to strength.

In the same fateful year that I discovered the letter, I was vaguely aware that she'd been awarded a Certificate of Merit (First Class) as Editor of the magazine by the British Association of Industrial Editors. So she was undoubtedly a serious player by that stage, and the magazine's team certainly involved some of the very best talent in Ireland. Full-colour 'Masterpieces of Painting' typically featured on the inside cover (the Summer 1962 edition contained a particularly poignant painting entitled *The Orphans*, by John Everett Millais), while the frontispiece was usually a bespoke composition reflecting the sometimes Pythonesque graphics of the day, or great Irish artists like Louis le Brocquy or Arthur Armstrong. During the 1960s, written contributions were made by up-and-coming newcomers like Flann O'Brien, Ulick O'Connor, Gerrit van Gelderen, Peter Somerville-Large, John B. Keane, Theodora FitzGibbon, and Michael Viney.

And the locations reached ranged far and wide, from St James' Gate to Nigeria and New York, as did the topics, from the activities of Guinness employees and their families to the economics and history of beer, preventive medicine in Trinity College's Moyne Institute, the Galway Oyster Festival and the Stradbally Steam Festival. Key to the success of the *Harp* was the extraordinary talent of the team my mother had managed to assemble around her. This included the photographer Tony O'Malley; Bernard Share, a writer of comic novels and later Editor of *Cara*, the Aer Lingus inflight magazine; Billy Bolger, a pioneering designer and illustrator; and Jarlath Hayes, one of Ireland's truly great graphic designers and designer of the Irish euro harp logo. All were extraordinary men who earned their glowing obituaries, and I revered them for their warm wit and exceptional talents. But I really loved their wonderful spouses. I didn't know it at the time but, with the wives – Maureen O'Malley in Cabinteely, Jill Share in Killiney, Eithne Bolger on Morehampton Terrace and, above all, the woman who was a surrogate mother to me, Oonagh Hayes in Stillorgan Grove – the team designed and delivered most of the happiest times of my childhood, as I rotated between their houses to be minded for hours, days or weeks at a time. I must also include, in this wives' network, Rita Quinn, in Dalkey, a friend of my mother from Wexford, and her husband, Bill, an ex-RAF navigator, military historian and a man who could turn his hand to almost any maintenance job in a house.

One day, I may learn the actual facts but, sadly, all the main protagonists are now dead, so my understanding of what happened in my early years is limited. It seems that, while I was in St Philomena's, my mother, Leslie and Doreen had devised a sort of strategy for me that involved a temporary placement in the orphanage until I was old enough to attend primary school, at which point I was brought home to live with my mother and sent to St Conleth's College, on Clyde Road, in Ballsbridge. The distinctively liberal St Conleth's, with its motto *Fide et Fortitudine* (faith and courage), proved to be ideally suited to the needs of an intensely nervous but curious and excitable youngster. I have never seen any proof, but I believe that Doreen Luke was the driving force behind my placement in St Conleth's, a move that I think was a perfect antidote to the effects of my complicated first few years. And in the decade I spent there, I went from orphanage boy to head boy. It was Doreen, too, who agreed that my birth certificate (issued in Hackney, in London, close to the London Hospital, where my mother was spirited by the Guinness 'family' to give birth in March 1959) should name me as 'Leslie Christopher Marshall Luke' (after my father and grandfather, the Marshall being my father's *nom de plume* as a writer).

For the woman who'd borne a half-dozen children to a man with this very name to endorse such a plan seems as unusual now as it must have been in 1959. And even when Leslie died in 1963 (suddenly, aged 48), for Doreen to have then 'adopted' me and my mother as a kind of personal charitable project still seems remarkable. Not only did she apparently plan what might be called a moderate success in terms of getting her husband's illegitimate offspring into polite society, she even monitored the little chap's progress, at least annually, when she took my mother and me out for afternoon tea in Dún Laoghaire, usually presenting me with a five-pound note or wallet to mark the occasion. So above all else, I remember Doreen's extraordinarily kindly demeanour, and even at this great distance, the word 'angel' always comes to mind when I think of her.

Half a century on, I can speculate as to why I was so shaken by the discovery of that letter, the brief but intense conversation with my mother and the revelation that 'Aunty' Doreen was my father's wife. I now think it was because, when I read its contents, I felt like a small boy with an awful lot to lose. And even if I couldn't make head nor tail of my life before I'd arrived in No. 33, the warm friendly world of the Hayes, Shares, next-door neighbours and other friends of my mother's was what I now knew and loved, so I couldn't bear the thought of being ejected from it. As far as I can recall, my sudden overwhelming feeling was a fear of having to return to the orphanage. And my secondary – and everlasting – response was that nothing was quite as it seemed.

Nowadays, the reaction to finding out that my parents weren't married would probably be, 'So what?' Back then, though, it wasn't so straightforward. And it wasn't really the revelation that my father had lived another life. Even by that stage I felt that he was an almost mythical figure, in an endlessly shifting narrative, to which my mother's friends kept adding.

'You're so like your dad!' they would say.

'Even down to the gestures,' others would add.

'And just as handsome,' winking at each other.

He'd been very charming, they agreed. I was 'the image'. And that's all they would say. But that had been enough, until then, because, while I had a very faint recollection of being with him, once, near a big car, like a Ford Zodiac, I'd only ever really seen him in a few photographs, in which he seemed to be rather nervously holding me when I was a toddler, smiling back, equally nervously.

No, the truth was that he inhabited a closed file in my consciousness, a file about which I was only curious because so many of my mother's girlfriends excitedly insisted that I was like a clone of my absent father. My main – my overriding – concern was my mother, not because of our fun-filled times together but because of the seemingly endless time we were apart. And because of all the sheer vagueness when it came to my father and St Philomena's. And because I was always being shunted between other mothers and houses. My mother was consistently tight-lipped about my father, so details were frustratingly hard to glean, no matter how often I would ask her. 'I don't know what to say,' she would reply to my earnest, even desperate, enquiries about my father over the decades. Towards the end of her life she did admit that Leslie had been the love of her life and that her heart had been completely broken when he died. But my heart almost broke when I heard that she'd burned all of his love letters to her, in 2002.

Her relative aversion towards discussing my father was as naught, however, when it came to the orphanage. On this issue she remained absolutely silent until she died. So it was only in her final years that I garnered a little information about my time in St Philomena's, and that was from my favourite 'other mother', Oonagh Hayes, when she came to stay with us in Cork once. The visit was unbeknownst to my real mother, so Oonagh could talk freely over a glass of wine in the kitchen. Oonagh was the only person who had any real idea of the reputation of the institution back in the 1960s. It was she who told me that I was 'handed over to the nuns' at such a young age, and she also recalled how one young nun, in particular, had 'adored' the small, dark and winsome 'little Christopher' and had actually quit the convent, distraught, after I left.

Oonagh believed that this had been a real blessing, having the love of at least one maternal figure while I was a little 'orphan'. She also recalled how she would sometimes visit my mother in No. 33 when my grandfather came to live with us in his final years, and how Christy would occasionally denounce his own daughter for her 'sinfulness'. He sometimes even declared, Oonagh said, that 'Colette has made her bed, and now she can lie in it'. Oonagh also recalled how once, when she asked him where I was, my grandfather quipped, 'The little b— is in his bedroom'. That was par for the course in those days in Ireland, I gather, and although I thought he was a cantankerous old man (whose pipe-smoking revolted me), I certainly never heard him use that term within my hearing. In any case, by the time Oonagh was revealing these unsavoury memories, I was pretty sure that I'd long since gotten over the whole thing, and I would just occasionally slip it into conversations to emphasise, perhaps, why my worldview wasn't always 'mainstream'.

It was only as I was flying to New York with my family, in 2016, that I abruptly began to appreciate the depths of my buried feelings about those early years, when I found myself quietly weeping at the end of the inflight movie, *Spotlight*.

This followed the story of the *Boston Globe* newspaper's Spotlight team, a famous investigative journalism unit, and their probe into the systemic child abuse in the Boston area by Roman Catholic priests. The parallels between Boston and Dublin, with knowledge of what was going on at the highest ecclesiastical level and the cover-up of a wickedness inflicted on generations of children by a few paedophile priests and their enablers, were unexpectedly sickening and appalling. The impact was worsened by the movie's epilogue, which informed viewers that Cardinal Law of Boston, who had presided over the whole affair, had actually been promoted to the Basilica di Santa Maria Maggiore in Rome.

Some months later, I plucked up the courage to watch the British film *Philomena*. This followed the course of another journalistic investigation into the case of Philomena Lee, who became pregnant when she was very young and was forced to give her baby son away to the nuns of Sean Ross Abbey, in County Tipperary, without a goodbye or even a clue as to his future. In fact, it transpired that, like so many illegitimate children in those 'orphanages', her son had been taken from his mother and promptly sold to an American couple for about £1,000. Eventually, Philomena and the journalist helping her, Martin Sixsmith, find out that her son, named Michael by his adoptive parents, had died of AIDS. But not long before he died, he had returned to Ireland to visit the Abbey, to learn more about his biological mother. In a devastating twist, the nuns told Michael that his mother had abandoned him and they had lost contact with her, when in fact they had forced her to sign an agreement never to make contact with her son again. In the end, after a 50-year quest, Philomena discovers that her son was actually buried in the Abbey's cemetery, but not before the one surviving nun who was involved tells the journalist that what had happened to Philomena and Michael was the result of her sexual sinfulness. In the final scenes, Martin is enraged by the nuns' behaviour, but Philomena prefers to forgive them. Again, alone on the couch at home, I welled up.

After my own mother died in 2019, I decided to undertake a little investigation of my own. This turned out to be shockingly simple, even though, for my own half-century, I'd never met anyone other than Oonagh who'd known about St Philomena's. So I was really taken aback when I typed the name into an online search engine and was instantly taken to a series of articles featuring the orphanage. The first was about an anonymised survivor:

Mary… had been born in St Patrick's Mother and Baby Home on the Navan Road and subsequently moved to St Philomena's Convent in Stillorgan, where she spent eight years, before she was subsequently moved to St Mary's Industrial School, in Sandymount. Mary was released on her 16th birthday, and she went to live with her mother, before being returned to St Philomena's a year later by her mother. Subsequently, she began to date a man that the nuns didn't like. One day, Mary found a policeman sitting in the parlour of the convent, and he escorted her to the Sisters of Our Lady of Charity Magdalene Laundry (commonly known as Gloucester Street), in Dublin. Mary tried to run away, but was caught and subsequently moved to the Good Shepherd Magdalene Laundry in Limerick where she spent nearly three years.

Another survivor, Christopher Neary, spent his childhood in a Church-run orphanage and an industrial school, but considers himself a 'very, very lucky man'. Christopher believes he is lucky to be alive. The 69-year-old recalls some devastating early memories of his time in St Philomena's. The nuns were harsh and they didn't like to hear the children in their care crying, he said. 'They gave me a black eye once and when I cried they told me if I didn't shut up the police would come and take me away,' he said. 'I also remember being pushed into a cupboard under the stairs.'

The third piece was in a report about another survivor, called Phyllis Morgan:

St Philomena's was a place run by a few sadistic nuns, very, very cruel you know, when you think – we were only children, four, five, six, seven, eight, nine, ten, you know – and you know, my young life was … this sense of fear all the time, waiting for the next beating … they used to beat us with hurling sticks … that … the workmen who done the painting and repairs around the convent … and the big farm had tapered the hurling stick so it just tapered down instead of that lumpy bit on the side. And you know that's what we used to get beaten with you know; you'd have to hold your hands out, you know, you were too terrified to be 'bold' as it was called … you'd think, 'my God is this nun ever gonna stop?' They'd be frothing at the mouth, you know, and … you'd be nearly fainting your hands would be so painful from the beatings …

Undoubtedly the most upsetting article I came across was by Liam Collins, in the *Irish Independent* in March 2017:

One of the convents was called St Philomena's; it was an orphanage run by a stern order of French nuns who all wore a huge, intimidating white bonnet, known, I believe, as a cornette. I can still remember, having robbed their orchard, looking behind as I fled down a tree-lined avenue, at the terrifying sight of one of these nuns bearing down on me. Just as she was about to seize me, I put on a spurt and escaped. Every Sunday we would watch, enthralled, as hundreds of young orphan boys marched silently out of what are now the gates of the Stillorgan Wood estate. They were graded according to height, and clad in identical suits, as they marched to the terminus of the number five bus for a weekly excursion. A group of us frequently sat on the wall watching this procession of 'the orphans' with a mixture of awe and apprehension.

Once, my mother, as she was coming along the road, stopped to talk to myself and my pals as we were observing the nuns and their charges, and, looking across as the boys were shepherded onto the bus, she remarked, 'I hope you realise how lucky you are!' Of course, I didn't.

Fifty years after I found that letter from my father, and fifty-five since I'd left St Philomena's, I found myself in a cold sweat reading the passage about 'young orphan boys' marching silently along the tree-lined drive from the main house at St Philomena's, instantly remembering – as I did with a terrifying vividness – the trees, that front gate, and those little boys, many of whom of course were not orphans at all. And one of them might have been me.

All this research may explain why I can recall so little of my earliest years. And why the letter, so trivial on its own, was significant only as a reminder of where I'd come from, and might *return* to. But turning that traumatic revelation on its head, looking back, as I now can, I am all the more certain that regardless of everything that followed those times, I was and I remain extraordinarily lucky.

I cannot honestly recall being beaten as a little boy in St Philomena's, but I do remember the suffocating, inescapable and perpetual dread I associated with the place. Reading others' memories of that fear provided an unexpected but welcome validation of my suppressed memories. Because it confirmed that I was not imagining things. I was not alone when it came to the fear, which had begun for me, and so many others, in the orphanage and had never really gone away.

Some people may find it hard to believe that an old emergency physician is driven by fear, but fear – or a free-floating anxiety anyway – has been a constant for me throughout my life. It has periodically swapped places with its twin sibling, anger, but mostly it has just hovered nearby. Oddly, I sometimes think of it now as a kind of gift that has drawn me towards others who are fearful, and has helped me to feel their pain, and – yes, sometimes angrily – motivated me to do something about it.

Mind Expanding

By the mid-seventies, within a few years of discovering the truth about my father, I had become one of those mildly crazy teenagers who are reckless, regularly in trouble at home and in school, and prone to romantic obsessions. It was in Amsterdam in 1976, however, that I discovered – painfully – what it's *really* like to lose your mind.

That was the year I did my Leaving Cert, at just seventeen years of age, and in the summer I travelled to the Continent with a few friends for an adventure that was every bit as fascinating and unforgettable as we'd been promised. After Paris, we'd headed to Amsterdam and camped in the city's immense Vondelpark, where, it was said, in that outpost of flower-power and hippies, 'everything is possible and [almost] everything is allowed'.

One evening, a quintessential hippy type turned up outside our tent, wearing a leather bus conductor's pouch, of a sort familiar to every passenger of a CIÉ bus in Dublin in the 1970s. Nervously glancing around, he'd lifted its flap and revealed, not a horde of greasy coins, but a bewildering range of packaged pills and powders for sale. As foolishly and unthinkingly as any seventeen-year-old young man who'd had a bottle or two of Dutch courage on a sunny evening in Amsterdam, I decided to try a tab of the 'acid' I'd been reading about that very year, in Aldous Huxley's *Doors of Perception* and Hunter S. Thompson's *Fear and Loathing in Las Vegas*.

Even if I had tried, it would have been very difficult in those pre-computer days to find the words to explain the hallucinatory effects of Lysergic acid diethylamide (LSD), which took an hour or so to kick in that night. But kick in they certainly did, and a couple of hours after placing a tiny blotting paper stamp impregnated with LSD on my tongue, I was in the throes of complete mental disintegration, rolling around inside the tent and on the grass outside, as everything in the world dissolved into a roiling multicoloured soup and spectacular jet-trails followed every aerial movement of my hands.

In hindsight, the primary sensation was what we now routinely call 'pixelation': a revelation that every normal image was actually composed of tiny spots or pixels of colour, which were as striking and unstable in my head that night as they must have seemed to people who saw them first on a *Top of the Pops* graphics display, or a frozen PC screen in the 1980s. Weirdly, sounds seemed to decompose too.

At that time, however, both pixels and sound droplets in one's head were entirely new, at least to a normally 'sane' young man, and I'm afraid that that trip to the park in Amsterdam turned out to be a very bad one indeed. I think I was actively hallucinating for at least twelve hours that night, and my world continued to shimmer and wobble vividly even as I insisted wildly to my companions that we must immediately flee the Vondelpark and hitch back to Paris on the main road south from the city. In fact, the intense fear and paranoia that engulfed me for those hours haunted me for months afterwards, in occasional flashbacks. Moreover, it took no effort at all in the decades that followed to believe that I'd a pretty good sense of what it truly meant to 'go mad'. The experience certainly convinced me that most people simply don't get what is meant by a so-called bad trip or a psychotic reaction to a drug.

Over the years since, when I've heard how others from my school and college days *never* fully recovered from their experimentation with LSD or other hallucinogens, I have felt the utmost pity and empathy for them. I think it also explains, to a large extent, why I've devoted so much of my career to highlighting the very real dangers of substance misuse, as well as poisoning in the broadest sense. Once bitten, and all that.

I cannot claim to have been totally transformed by this experience when I got back to Dublin (the delicious beer in Belgium provided appropriate relief in the immediate aftermath), but I'm fairly sure it featured subconsciously in my eventual career choice. That decision was fiendishly simple: Law or Medicine. My mother, although fiercely supportive of my general educational progress, was reluctant to steer me in any particular direction, and so it was that that summer, in the midst of the 1976 heatwave, I found myself sitting on the grassy bank outside the old Stillorgan Post Office, juggling offers and applications for Medicine in UCD and Law at Trinity College.

Genuinely unsure as to which to choose, I sat there for an hour or so, engaged in a particularly intense debate with myself about the pros and cons of a career in either of the two ancient professions. 'Gravitas, wig and gown' topped the list for Law, while 'doing some good' and my enthusiasm for the TV medics of *M*A*S*H* made the case for Medicine.

Looking back now, I may also have had notions about the 'power of compassion' for others versus the 'might of legal rhetoric' put into my head by two particularly brilliant teachers at my school, St Conleth's, in Ballsbridge. And, on mature reflection, it was probably one of many quips I'd filed away during Michael Gardiner's English classes that nudged me in one direction. 'Lawyers, I suppose, were children once,' he said, quoting the view of William Hazlitt, the great English essayist, after an unhappy legal encounter. And then there was the oft-alleged distinction between the two professions, learned in the legally trained Peter Gallagher's often uproarious history classes: 'Lawyers rob you, sure, but doctors rob you, and then they *kill* you'. As usual, humour clinched it for me.

A final factor that may well have influenced my decision, although I wasn't conscious of it outside the Post Office that day, was the Oil Crisis of 1973, when Arab states hostile to Israel raised oil prices by up to 300 per cent in punitive measures aimed at countries deemed to be Israel's main supporters, like the UK and USA. This led to massive price hikes, fuel shortages and generalised economic misery throughout the West, and Ireland was not spared. In fact, my own poor mother had lost her so-called job-for-life due to cutbacks in Guinness, where she worked in the Press Office, and many of her friends were also struggling to pay mortgages and school fees, as cutbacks, bank strikes and economic incompetence blighted the lives of most people here. Worse still, by the late 1970s, Ireland had acquired a reputation internationally as the economic 'sick man of Europe'. For me, in the end, the security of Medicine – and the distinctly dreamy possibility of doing good – trumped the cachet of Law. So into the postbox went my letter to the Medical School at UCD. I received my letter of acceptance a couple of weeks later and, by September 1976, I was officially a medical student, starting the re-Medicine year in UCD.

One of the many things that secondary school doesn't prepare you for is the sometimes shocking mismatch between a school-leaver's expectations and the reality of undergraduate life in university. So when I arrived for my first day as a Pre-Med in the Science Building on UCD's Belfield site, between Donnybrook and Stillorgan, I was entirely unprepared for the vast concrete jungle that I found on the newish campus. The science block itself, one of the oldest buildings in Belfield, and the location of lectures for the most junior medical, dental and veterinary undergraduates, was a particularly unattractive construction, with a blend of wood, concrete and glass that resembled the unlovely Hawkins House on the corner of Poolbeg Street, in Dublin's city centre, which was for a long time the address of the Department of Health.

The other neophytes in its main auditorium on our first day struck me as mostly earnest and straitlaced types, who had clustered keenly in the lower tiers, close to the lectern, while I snuck in the back door to take what was to become my preferred discreet position in the penny seats. And then, like some pantomime figure, the legendary Professor Carmel Humphries suddenly appeared in her black robe, shushed the assembled multitude of pre-meds, pre-dents and pre-vets and, her eyes swivelling upwards, uttered some memorable but not terribly reassuring words of welcome:

'Ah yes, the cream of the country – rich and thick!' Already as nervous as anyone else in the audience, I was taken aback by that Beckettian reference from the brilliant zoologist. I glanced sideways with a nervous smirk (meaning 'Yikes!') at my newest acquaintance, Audoen Healy, who'd sat down beside me in the back row moments before, still clad in his bomber command jacket, huge boots and full-face motorbike helmet.

We both inhaled deeply, shook our heads in mock outrage and laughed.

I said, 'Jeez, that's some introduction!'

He nodded vigorously and grinned, but didn't disagree.

And so began our undergraduate careers.

Although I subsequently learned that Professor Humphries had a famously wry sense of humour, and her lectures were typically colourful, her introductory sarcasm had seriously punctured my highly inflated version of medical school. Within a few weeks, I found myself disillusioned and disappointed with life in the science building. I struggled with Physics, which I hadn't studied in school, and Biochemistry. It wasn't that I didn't see the point of them, it was just that they were so hard, and the whole Pre-Med experience seemed so desperately *dull*.

Homesick for school and missing the routines of old friendships, I increasingly drifted towards the Arts building and the Student Bar, in search of someone with whom to discuss the Big Ideas that I thought were the point of university education. The Bar became my base camp for that year, as I made friends with undergraduates who were reading English, French, Economics, Politics and History. Anything, in fact, other than Biochemistry and Physics.

I also made a concerted effort to locate the much-vaunted pleasures of college. I joined DramSoc, in the legendary LG1 basement theatre space, and it was here that I spent much of that first year, with future stalwarts of Irish theatre, like Gerry Stembridge, Ben Barnes, Mary Ryan, John Meaney, and Michael Scott. I played tennis with my other new best friend, Declan Sheerin, tried a little (Thirds) rugby and I even found myself bowling for UCD in Stillorgan. And I accidentally joined the winning side in that year's campus campaign for presidency of the Students' Union, won by Conall O Morain. Ironically, I later came to be an admirer of the losing candidate, Fintan O'Toole, who remains one of my favourite 'agitators' in the country. However, Conall had asked me first, and I was too polite to say no. The last I heard, Fintan didn't do too badly in the end.

Notwithstanding these extracurricular pursuits, live music was my favourite team activity, and the main agenda item each week was the Saturday night concert in the main canteen on the top floor of the Arts block in Belfield. Although run pretty amateurishly by the UCD Students' Union, this was a hugely popular event in the social life of Dublin in the mid-1970s and attracted hundreds of young people, mostly students, to one of the few enclosed spaces in the city then capable of accommodating big crowds to see the likes of Supply, Demand and Curve, Louis Stewart, Freddie White, Elvis Costello and my own favourites, Alberto y Los Trios Paranoias.

In spite of my determined socialising, that first year was an emotional rollercoaster as I adjusted to a new life seeing a lot less of my old gang, dialling down an intense teenage romance with my long-term girlfriend, Kathy Noone in Glenageary, and struggling to adapt to a course that seemed difficult and dreary in contrast with life in the Arts building. At night, despite the joys of LG1, the tennis courts or the Bar, life in Belfield tended to wind down after 6.00 p.m., and I'd often go home on the crowded rush-hour bus, alone and despondent. Worse still, when it came to my academic progress, I started to experience an entirely new phenomenon: failing, and having to repeat, exams.

Looking back, I felt too young for college, abandoned by the university system, and crushed by the loss of close school friendships and the clearly terminal stages of my relationship with Kathy. Erratic weekend rendezvous with the lads didn't compensate for the many hours of close contact we'd had in the school years and, to make matters worse, my closest schoolfriends, like Ray Victory, David O'Donohoe, Peter Kenny, Mark O'Donovan and Damian Neylin, were all now scattered in different third-level institutions, so our once-fraternal relationships were abruptly diminished. Just as painfully, but more unexpectedly, one of the other people I really cared about, John Larchet, a classmate since the 1960s and jester-in-chief in our little gang, stood up abruptly one night in the Queens pub in Dalkey and announced that he'd had 'enough' of our endless search for suburban parties and dull evenings in the pub, and he stormed off, almost never to be seen again.

I did my best to reconnect with John when I was in Australia a decade later, as did the other guys over the years, but he basically gave us the runaround. The closest I got to seeing him again in person was in the hearse containing his ashes at his funeral in Donnybrook in 2016, when a half-dozen of his school and college friends sat scattered about the back of an almost-empty church, while his heartbroken family grieved in the front pew, including the young son and partner he'd left behind. John came from one of Dublin's most famous musical and artistic families and was a namesake of his grandfather, a celebrated composer and Professor of Music in UCD. He was also one of the most charismatic people I've ever known, always fizzing with energy and surreal notions. In retrospect, alas, it was probably predictable that he would rise to the top of Saatchi & Saatchi in Sydney, then become bored and retrain as a wine connoisseur in the States and Europe.

Outside the church that afternoon, reassembling the story of his life from the snippets offered by grieving siblings and former friends, it seems that John had spent his life constantly moving on, from location to location, relationship to relationship, until he succumbed to the years of fast living. The tragedy was that he was so loved by all who came into his orbit, but he broke many hearts on the way, including those of his school friends in 1976. In the following 40 years, his was possibly the first funeral at which I remained dry-eyed.

For me, the drudgery of the study and the disillusionment with the life of a medical student were intense, and I came close on several occasions to leaving for a more enjoyable or interesting course. But it was people, as always, who rescued me from my slough of despond, and as my school friends drifted away, it was my new college friends who buoyed me up. In any event, my Pre-Med year eventually petered out, and I scraped into First Med, after repeating one or two tests in the summer of 1977. It was a heck of a comedown from school academic gold medallist to glad-just-to-pass, but my heart wasn't in it, and I suspect it was only the potential shame I attached to the idea of dropping out that propelled me forward.

First Med kicked off in autumn 1977 and seemed somehow easier, even if it was mainly because we 'medics' moved into town, to the medical school in Earlsfort Terrace. Originally built for the Dublin International Exhibition of Arts and Manufacture, or Great Exhibition, in 1865, the Terrace had been the massive main building of UCD since 1908. Back in 1977, it was an impressive grey building containing the Medical School, with the Anatomy Department at the back on the Hatch Street side, located beside the School of Architecture, with Physiotherapy, the Medical School offices and sundry other lecture theatres on the other side, and the *Aula Maxima* in the middle. The Aula was the great hall where we did our exams that year (it was later converted into the National Concert Hall, which opened in 1981).

By the late 1970s, the place was jaded and a little shabby, with broken Victorian fittings and rude graffiti aplenty. The Anatomy Department, where we had our main morning lectures, contained an ancient wooden theatre, and the Dissecting Room, with its stinking baths full of formaldehyde embalming mixtures, was next door. My enduring memory of that year is of the choking tang of formaldehyde and the grey flesh of elderly cadavers as each week a little group assigned to each body took it in turns to dissect a limb, torso, head or neck. And, yes, like most of my classmates, I was probably shaking slightly when we were first brought into the room and the draped cadavers were finally revealed to us.

I found the dissection lessons were hindered by an inescapable nausea, provoked by the fluid and the flesh. Still, there is no doubt that the black medical humour many of us were to deploy in our subsequent careers was first developed in that Dissecting Room and, the longer we stood around the tables, the queasier and giddier we tended to get.

In hindsight, my mixed feelings about a career in medicine weren't much helped by the Anatomy lessons, or the associated Edwardian textbooks. And the desperately dull lectures in Physiology were a complete passion-killer. Consequently, my enthusiasm remained at a low ebb, so my typical day in 1977 started late, outside the Anatomy Department, where I would arrive at around 10.30 a.m. for the 9.00 a.m. start, and rendezvous with two other new friends, Tommy and Kieran, who were also night owls, with the same habit of sleeping in. Invariably, like the bored vultures in *The Jungle Book*, our first agenda item was: 'So what we gonna do?' The usual response: 'I dunno. What d'you wanna do?' More often than not we would head for coffee or, if we were exceptionally late, an early lunch in Hartigan's, on Leeson Street, the meeting place favoured by the Medical and Engineering students of UCD since time immemorial.

Like every good pub, Harto's had a regular clientele, which included students of different classes as well as their lecturers, some of whom spent even more time at the bar than the most bibulous of their students. Our (vulture-like) strategy back then was to wait for the more studious of Harto's undergraduate regulars to come over for their lunch and pump them for a summary of the morning's Anatomy and Physiology lectures. Remarkably, this worked for a while, which meant there was more time to wander through St Stephen's Green to Dawson Street and Nassau Street, where it was possible to spend a happy hour or two in the warmth of a bookshop. Or I might head to Grafton Street, where I worked in the evenings as a kitchen porter in Captain America's (and, later, its sister restaurant, Solomon Grundy's on Suffolk Street). Or sometimes I would just wander along Grafton Street until I bumped into a passing acquaintance and we might head for a pint in Kehoes or The Bailey. Looking back, these were relatively blissful days, when a crammer like me could get by, in the absence of a continuous assessment system, by studying late at night and picking the brains of cleverer colleagues.

The next few years in Earlsfort Terrace flew by in what now seems like a pleasant daze. Sadly, I was 'let go' by Kathy, but I found compensatory friendship and affection with a growing number of medical school classmates who succeeded in luring me into the Terrace for social reasons if nothing else. And even if I wasn't what one might call a model medical student, I was hardworking in my own way. I studied the relevant medical books, when I could, and although my exam results were routinely borderline, they were enough to sustain a forward momentum.

One of the advantages of an unusually long undergraduate career – six years in the case of medical students – was the number and variety of adventures that it made possible. For me, these included working holidays in Dutch and German factories, after the bar and restaurant work of term time, sun holidays in Ios and Giglio (of *Concordia* shipwreck fame), expeditions to music festivals in Reading, Saarbrücken, Lisdoonvarna and Dalymount, as well as brief group trips around Ireland. The best of these staycations involved country house parties in North County Dublin, holiday cottages in West Cork, Jazz weekends in Cork and Sligo, and a quest for the source of the River Shannon. And in those youthful days, every adventure seemed to have at least one 'episode'.

This ranged from sleeping rough under the stage at the Sligo Jazz Festival tent, after the legendary Acker Bilk had finished his set, to contending with a close friend who was behaving more and more oddly in our rented cottage (and the pub, and eventually on the street), and who sadly turned out to be having an acute psychotic episode. This, in hindsight, explained some of his previous eccentric activities, and it was a tragic forerunner of an illness that was to be pretty disabling. And he wasn't the only one. I think there were more than a few in my class who developed severe mental illness during their first twelve months after qualifying. And there was at least one death that I heard was attributed to suicide on the stairwell in the Terrace.

One of the most unforgettable nights of my own medical student days was when I was working one night as a kitchen porter in Captain America's restaurant, and the roof above the main oven caught fire. Normally the chirpy and very cool chef would squirt the frequent flames at the back of his oven with a fire extinguisher and that would be that, but for some miraculous reason, on this occasion, he suddenly roared, 'Everyone get out!!! Now!!' Minutes later the ceiling imploded in flames just a few feet away from me as I made good my escape.

Happily, although it was a close call, no one was significantly injured in the fire, and the kitchen crew and front-of-house staff went on afterwards to have one of the best parties (or wakes) I've ever been at. And I've always thought that that chef should have received a medal for saving numerous lives that evening.

This was in stark contrast to another event that has also stayed with me ever since. This happened while a small gang of us, including myself and my great undergraduate friends in UCD, David Valentine and Hugh Comerford, were amusing ourselves in remotest County Leitrim by searching for the source of the Shannon, on St Valentine's Day in 1981. We had stopped for a pub lunch in Ballinamore, about a half-hour's drive from the Shannon Pot, when news of the *Stardust* nightclub disaster began to percolate through on the radio. I remember being transfixed by the emerging story of so many youngsters dying in a massive conflagration at the nightclub, in Artane in Dublin, where just a few weeks before some of my own school friends had been at a concert.

Of course, in those days we were all relatively frequent visitors to the city-centre clubs in Leeson Street or Harcourt Street, and even to far-flung places like Tamangos in Portmarnock or the Pierre in Dún Laoghaire. So it didn't take much imagination to envisage the mass panic that must have taken hold when the lights in the main *Stardust* dance area went out as the fire enveloped the electricity circuits. Reports afterwards described how the ceiling began to melt onto clubbers (huge drums of cooking oil had been stored on the first floor), and people were trampled on as they tried desperately to escape through exits that led into toilets or were blocked by metal bars, chained tables and steel plates that even the fire engines couldn't budge. In total, 48 young people died as a result of the inferno that night, half of them eighteen years old or younger. A further 214 were injured, and five weren't identified until suitable DNA technology became available in 2007. It was probably the most shocking episode of my youth, after the Dublin and Monaghan bombings of 1974.

For all my meandering ways, I finally got fired up about Medicine as a career when we reached the so-called clinical, or bedside, years of medical school. This happened from Fourth Year on, when we were despatched to various hospitals to work on the ground. For me, this meant St Vincent's Hospital in Elm Park, Saint John of God's in Stillorgan, the Coombe Maternity Hospital and the Mater Hospital in Dublin, and Monaghan General Hospital, to see what actually happened in the wards, clinics, labour suites and operating theatres. In short, we left behind the dreary theory, and often drearier lectures in the Terrace, for the real world.

Given that I spent much of the first half of medical school working in another world, albeit of pubs, kitchens and factories, and as little time as possible in the medical school library, I was pleasantly surprised to be captivated by the very real stories of patients and by the medical and nursing practice I saw in front of me. This included the general surgery and medicine of the county hospital, the sometimes intractable psychoses or melancholia of the psychiatric institution, and the vast range of medical and surgical presentations in teaching hospitals on both sides of the Liffey. Equally important, we finally met practising professionals, as opposed to sometimes reluctant or soporific academics who made it plain that they preferred the armchairs of the Royal College or the barstool of Harto's to the lecterns of the Terrace. It was a revelation to see how some doctors or nurses could be rock stars as much as their TV, music or literary counterparts. And it is remarkable how even a brief exposure to some of these surgeons, physicians, psychiatrists and nurses inspired a lifelong admiration.

I particularly remember undertaking a surgical attachment in St Vincent's in Dublin, which was my base hospital, and unexpectedly finding myself one lunchtime in the passenger seat of Professor Niall O'Higgins' sports car, hurrying to the National Maternity Hospital in Holles Street to undertake an emergency appendicectomy in a pregnant woman. I think the fact that I'd already survived several hours assisting him in the operating theatre in St Vincent's had persuaded the eminent surgeon to suggest that I 'come along for the ride' to the obstetric hospital to assist him there.

To this day, I remember the boyish thrill of rushing from one hospital to another to perform what was a potentially critical operation as an emergency. The journey to the city centre was exhilarating enough for a medical student who'd never really been up close to a surgeon before, never mind the future President of the Royal College of Surgeons of Ireland, but my driver's intense concentration and unwavering focus, moving swiftly from the breast surgery list in Elm Park to an urgent emergency procedure in Holles Street, was so zen-like that it was etched indelibly in my brain. The surgery itself was swift and unremarkable, as it so often is, aside from the gravid uterus that had to be negotiated, but the sheer excitement of that micro-adventure meant that I entertained the notion of a surgical career for a few years afterwards. And I remained a fanboy of Professor O'Higgins for the rest of my medical life.

Undoubtedly, the greatest adventure of my medical school years was a trip to Zambia to undertake a six-week elective stint in 1981, in Monze mission hospital, about 200 kilometres south of the capital, Lusaka. The hospital had been run since 1976 by Sister Lucy O'Brien, a celebrated Irish missionary and surgeon-obstetrician who had qualified in UCD in 1952, undertaken obstetric training in London and Bristol, and had already done trojan work in Biafra and Sierra Leone before moving permanently to Zambia.

I travelled to Southern Africa with a classmate, Catherine Stuart, under the auspices of the UCD version of the VSO (Voluntary Service Overseas) development charity, whose mission was 'to create lasting change through volunteering'. And it has to be said that there really wasn't a dull moment in the entire expedition, from the moment we nearly missed our Aeroflot flight as we scoured the duty-free shops in Heathrow, to being initially denied access to the connecting flight in Moscow, then travelling on a series of terrifyingly shaky Russian planes full of KGB agents (we suspected) sitting in every third row, in identical green or brown suits. Notwithstanding the stress of the attempted scam in Moscow airport – where they demanded cash to allow us to continue our travel, resulting in a mildly riotous rush for the next flight – we arrived in a bombed-out airport in Luanda, in Angola, where a civil war was clearly in progress, with Soviet and Cuban personnel and material discernible about the hangars and runways.

Eventually, thoroughly disabused of the joy of air travel, we reached Lusaka airport and with remarkably little fuss travelled down the largely unmarked main road to the mission hospital in Monze. This was a simple affair, comprising a collection of single-storey buildings and what seemed to be plenty of car-parking space out front. In fact, this turned out to be where hundreds of hopeful patients congregated on weekdays. The hospital was situated across the road from an outdoor market selling ebony and ivory carvings, and a small supermarket, whose shelves remained almost bare for the duration of our time in the little town, aside from a few bits of meat, local vegetables and hardware. This was a sign of the hard economic times in that once prosperous maize-growing part of Zambia, but we two students were relatively comfortably accommodated in a guest bungalow in the hospital compound, in humbling contrast to the local populace, most of whom lived in grass huts.

Zambia was originally part of the colonial Central African Federation and was called Northern Rhodesia: with Southern Rhodesia (which became Zimbabwe in 1980), it had once been the 'breadbasket' of Southern Africa, and it also supplied much of the world's copper. However, after independence in 1964, the economy had slowly crumbled, as the Soviet Union flooded global markets with copper, the 1973 Oil Crisis took hold, and Zambia became embroiled in a series of Southern African wars of independence. The Rhodesians periodically bombed or raided encampments of Zimbabwean and Namibian rebel movements within the country, while the African National Congress had their exile headquarters in Lusaka. By 1981, when we arrived there, Zambia was largely dependent on subsidies from sympathetic countries like China, Russia, Yugoslavia and Scandinavia. Nonetheless, my abiding memory of the country is of the gentle nature of its people and their stoicism in the face of what seemed to us soft Europeans to be serious privation.

If my initial exposure to bedside medicine in Dublin had been a revelation, then those few weeks in Monze were an unforgettable immersion in industrial amounts of surgery, obstetrics and medicine. The hospital, which had begun as a small health clinic in the early 1960s, had been developed and modernised by Sr O'Brien and it genuinely did cater for Anything & Everything. Particularly novel local pathology included severe bites by hippopotami (these volatile inhabitants of local rivers seemed to enjoy overturning boatloads of humans and mauling them, often lethally), trachoma (a painful eye infection that often causes blindness in those without access to medication and ophthalmic surgery), huge levels of tuberculosis and, one of the perennial problems in Africa, obstetric fistula (a tear in the birth canal due to difficult childbirth), causing incontinence and misery for many childbearing women. In fact, Sr O'Brien's success in treating such fistulae led to Monze being named subsequently as the National Fistula Centre for Zambia.

Catherine and I joined the medical and nursing teams on their ward rounds, and we encountered a huge variety of pathology that would rarely have been seen in Ireland. This often meant we got involved in all sorts of medical procedures, including my first pericardiocentesis (using a very large needle to drain thick, tubercular pus from around the heart) in a patient with advanced TB. We also saw, for the first time and close up, patients with intractable leprosy or albinism who were largely ostracised in the community. And, of course, we had the immense privilege of assisting Sr O'Brien and her colleagues in a wide range of trauma cases, abdominal and gynaecological operations, and deliveries in the labour ward, so that by the end of the elective, any nervousness about clinical practice was largely banished. Firstly, we got to 'open' and 'stitch' and to handle anatomy in the midst of such procedures. Secondly, we saw the impact of the calm and courteous approach of Sr O'Brien in the operating theatre, which was in stark contrast to many of her counterparts in this country. And thirdly, we learned about the economics of surgery on a shoestring.

This was where I first saw ultraviolet light – in the form of sunlight – being used to sterilise operating theatre drapes and gowns, which were hung over the hedges outside the hospital after their use in theatre each day. In short, nothing was wasted, and I have never seen a more environmentally aware and sustainable type of medical practice.

The stint in Monze was profoundly influential upon my career, even if I was not immediately aware of it at the time. I think if I was to identify a single reason for this, it would be that I was completely converted to the concept of 'needs must' and *doing the most good to the most people in the most need* (a phrase coined by the Salvation Army's Evangeline Booth during World War I, which later became a key tenet of emergency medicine in the twentieth century).

The trip was a revelation in other ways, too, with our forays into the town and brief excursions about its perimeter, and every night we were surprised by the beautiful, abrupt sunsets. And occasionally we were allowed to borrow a hospital Land Rover to explore the local area. (To this day, I regret that one such trip led to a stone cracking the windscreen as we hurtled though some woodland.)

Once a fortnight, Catherine and I would get a lift to Lusaka from a young Finnish agronomist, in his sleek white Mercedes estate. This luxurious, air-conditioned vehicle offered a stark contrast to the very basic provisions in the hospital, but not as much as the gated Scandinavian compound in Lusaka, where we entered a proto-IKEA interior world of platinum blonde children, elegant pine furniture and delicious coffee, served with dainty biscuits in charming crockery. This Friday afternoon delight was not enough, however, for our driver, who would spend the first half of the weekend unburdening himself of his deep-seated melancholia and angst. So severe was his unhappiness, indeed, that for years I came to imagine Finland as being like Ireland in the 1950s, a place of colonial oppression and post-colonial depression. In our case, it was the British Empire, in theirs, it was Swedish expansionism, but the impact was apparently the same.

In fact, our Finnish friend had a very severe dose of disillusionment. He explained that he was an agronomist involved in teaching trainees in an agricultural college near Monze, which had been funded by the Labour Party in Helsinki. His party was very sympathetic to the 'African socialism' of Zambia's essentially autocratic President Kaunda, he said, and it sent millions of dollars annually to Lusaka in aid. But, according to our friend, a huge proportion of this was 'siphoned off' in the airport to various ministers and their friends, and the melancholic Finn was terminally disenchanted with the whole business.

Indeed, nothing would do for him but to self-medicate with a huge dose of beer and vodka every other Friday night and go night-clubbing in downtown Lusaka. And, if nothing else, there was for us two medical students the compensation of seeing so many Zambians forgetting their worries, at least for a night, and dancing to their hearts' content. In addition to the local travel, Catherine and I travelled to Malawi, and I recall paddling in the shallow waters of Lake Malawi, the fifth-largest lake in the world. This was regarded then as a little dangerous due to the risk of acquiring bilharziasis or schistosomiasis, an unpleasant disease of the bladder, kidneys and liver that can be caught from larvae released from freshwater snails in the lake. In the early 1980s transmission was rare, but subsequent overfishing meant that the snails multiplied and the rates of the disease in Malawi have rocketed.

The other memorable feature of that trip to Malawi was the 750-kilometre journey from the capital, Lilongwe, back to Lusaka, on a crowded bus that stopped at one point in the middle of the bush, 'for passengers' refreshment'. We were all led to a nearby hamlet to sample some of the local beer, that looked and tasted like a muddy broth containing bits of grass. Thankfully, it wasn't comparable with the notorious ayahuasca drink of South America and, once the bitterness and bits were disregarded, the effect was quite soothing for the rest of a very bumpy journey home.

We also travelled to Zimbabwe, which in 1981 was in its first year of post-colonial and post-civil war independence under the rule of President Robert Mugabe. I recall how we were both amazed by the Toytown perfection of the roads and little towns once we'd crossed the Zambian border at Kariba. The capital, Harare, looked much more Anglo than Lusaka, while the hotels and collected buildings near Victoria Falls were the quintessence of British Empire style, circa 1900. And, of course, the Falls themselves and the safari park we briefly visited, in Hwange, were spectacular, in the way of so much of the enormous continent.

I'll never forget the return journey from Africa, again on juddering Aeroflot planes, back the way we came, with just one misadventure, when Catherine and I found ourselves in an army jeep in an Eastern European airport, chasing a taxiing plane, which stopped so that two very agitated Irish students could clamber aboard and get home. I confess that I developed an acute aversion to flying after that trip, which wasn't helped by the crash of another Aeroflot flight to Sierra

Leone, in July 1982, which killed all 90 occupants, including, I believe, Irish medical students en route to their medical electives.

I also had a recurrent paranoia that I'd definitely acquired schistosomiasis, a niggling belief that was only cured years later when I learned that the risk had only become significant in the mid-1980s. Notwithstanding the acquired distaste for air travel, an important legacy of my trip to Monze was a vital dose of growing up, as well as an aspiration to undertake some sort of altruistic or missionary medicine once I'd qualified. I was also finally cured of the sort of simplistic student politics that had taken hold of me briefly during my weekly 'tutorials' with Hugh Comerford in Doheny & Nesbitt's pub, on Baggot Street in Dublin, when I believed very briefly that some kind of utopian socialism might be the cure to the woes of Africa.

In fact, the corruption, economic mismanagement and endless civil wars I came to think were endemic in many parts of Southern Africa put an end to any notion that an -*ism* (communism, socialism, fascism, etc.) was the solution to anything. In truth, I was much more radicalised by exposure to the vast reality of poverty, the self-service synonymous with so many -*isms* and (although we only learned of it later) the horror of civil and tribal warfare that was going on in Zimbabwe even as we visited the nearby tourist sites. In 1981, then, I was convinced forever of the supremacy of compassion, above all other political belief systems. And, certainly, for the entirety of my career, I have thought of the diminutive Sr Lucy as one of the few truly iconic *and* heroic surgeons and teachers it has been my privilege to know.

One of the most important life lessons I learned in the final years of medical school was that the devil you know generally *is* better than the devil you don't know. This often uncomfortable lesson was so relevant that I was taught it twice in my final year.

Lesson No. 1 was obstetric. My formal training in the subject had taken place in the Coombe hospital, near Dolphin's Barn, and I'd really enjoyed this attachment in that part of Dublin, near my mother's former workplace in St James' Gate and my grandfather's childhood home. However, during my time in the Zambian labour wards, I had been inspired by one particular book, *The Active Management of Labour*, written by Professor Kieran O'Driscoll, former Master of the Coombe's great rival institution, the National Maternity Hospital, in Holles Street. O'Driscoll had initiated a quiet revolution in care in the delivery suite in the 1960s, aimed at reducing maternal mortality through education, organisation and communication around every aspect of labour, especially in first pregnancies. And I was really taken by this slim publication, which was set out in a refreshingly novel way. Each chapter started with an outline of the educational aims of the following few pages and closed with a reiteration of the lessons within the chapter.

The following chapter did the same, but first recapped what had been set out in the previous chapter. The book also employed simple diagrams, like the so-called partogram, a graphic colour-coded representation of the timeline of a delivery. This all sounds like a blindingly obvious structure nowadays, but in my undergraduate days, dense, dreary and sometimes Victorian textbooks were the norm, and it was a penitential exercise trying to read many of them. In contrast, *Active Management* communicated its key ideas in a strikingly clear and memorable manner. In a nutshell, the aim was to conclude a woman's first labour within twelve hours, inducing labour if necessary with a nick in the amniotic sac – the membranous bag around the baby – using a crochet-hook-like amnihook; the labour process was then to be monitored carefully by midwives and obstetricians, with measurement of the dilatation of the cervical *os* (opening); an accelerant, oxytocin, could be infused in cases of marked delay to try to amplify uterine contractions, and Pethidine could also be administered in calibrated 'aliquots' for pain, as necessary. According to Professor O'Driscoll, the aim of the process was to bring a 'military precision' to the organisation and monitoring of labour. His prescription had an enormous impact on obstetric practice in Ireland for decades afterwards, and it was recommended in a WHO bulletin as recently as 2009.

The problem for me was that, while I was an eager convert to O'Driscoll's Holles Street method, when I came to my final-year Obstetrics and Gynaecology *Viva* in Newman House (the nucleus of the original UCD on St Stephen's Green, now housing the Museum of Literature in Ireland), I found myself like piggy-in-the-middle between two giants of the rival Coombe and National Maternity Hospitals. I could clearly see and hear the mounting irritation of the Coombe Master, the lead interrogator, as I insisted on giving answers to each of his questions about labour in the Holles Street method, which was clearly not to the taste of the Coombe chief at that time. Simultaneously, I was trying not to add too obviously to the quiet satisfaction plainly visible on Professor O'Driscoll's face.

It was a highly risky tactic, this potential slighting of a hospital consultant, and a powerful Master in his own right, and one that could have landed a medical student in the proverbial. It is a trap into which I was later to fall, heavily, but on this occasion, I got away with it, and I squeezed past the Final Obstetrics hurdle, having gambled that O'Driscoll was still the better ally, politically.

Lesson No. 2 was paediatric. Again, it involved a *Viva* exam in my final year, when I found myself on the neonatal ward in Temple Street Children's Hospital, awaiting my turn in the Final Paediatric clinical exam.

Having had a sleepless night due to a cocktail of last-minute cramming and nerves, I was almost faint with fatigue, but my stress and adrenaline levels soared when the kindly invigilator beckoned me forward into a long ward, lined with windowed cubicles on both sides, and asked, 'Would you prefer Professor O'Doherty or Professor O'Donohoe?', probably expecting me to say that I didn't mind. What she couldn't have known was that, just a few days previously, Niall O'Donohoe, the eminent paediatric neurologist and Trinity professor, had politely suggested that I leave his home. Not because I was a dangerous intruder, but because I was one of his sons' closest friends and there had been an episode of irrational youthful exuberance at an impromptu gathering in his Dartry dwelling which had disturbed his important work in the study. I had been very embarrassed by the collective eviction, and I certainly wasn't ready to meet the good professor again quite so soon.

On the other hand, Professor Niall O'Doherty, another globally renowned paediatrician, was someone I was just as anxious not to meet that morning, given his legendary volatile disposition. So after a few moments of agonising reflection, I took a high-risk punt and said to the invigilator, 'I'll take Prof O'Donohoe, please.' I've never regretted that decision, although years later it was added to a long list of reasons to call me the thin ice-skating champion of the world. The Prof, as I knew him until he died recently, knocked on the glass door of the neonatal cubicle before coming in and saying, in a barely audible whisper, 'Good morning, Chris. Now, would you like to tell me what you have found with this baby?'

To this day, I've no idea what was wrong with that infant, aside from some kind of viral rash, but the professionalism of the Prof was a revelation. Kindness personified, domestic prejudices suspended, he ignored my nervous exhaustion and nursed me through the interrogation process until I escaped, extremely lightly, from the ward a half-hour later. The other, written parts of the Paediatric exams went reasonably well after that, and I passed that penultimate test before my Final Medical exams the following summer. In due course, I learned that Professor O'Doherty had failed almost everybody on his side of the ward that day, and they'd all had to repeat their Paediatric finals. For my part, that was another narrow escape, and never forgotten.

By that time, I was getting the hang of the medical student thing, at long last, so for the first time in six undergraduate years, there were no more major mishaps, no more than the usual distractions, and no further delay in obtaining my new post-nominal letters, which meant I could legally call myself, Dr C. Luke MB BCh BAO. I won't deny that that was a bit of a thrill after all the years of uncertain progress.

And looking back, now, I suddenly recall that on the UCD medics' graduation day in June 1982, my mother was in her early sixties, precisely the same age as I am now. For my part, I am blessed with four children, and a wife, while my unmarried mother had but one troublesome offspring. I distinctly remember the pride on her face on that sunny graduation day in Belfield. She had *always* believed in me, I knew, but it can't have been easy watching her crazy son skating out on that thin ice for so long.

The Yellow Pack Doctor

The exhausting blur of the final years of medical school, with the constant exam stress, eventually came to an end in the summer of 1982 when, in spite of myself, I qualified as a doctor. No honours were involved, I had nothing whatsoever to brag about, and the key to my modest success was the highly 'flexible' training available at University College Dublin. Still, I'd survived the climb. There was one last hedonistic fling, when a gang of us final meds stayed above a pizzeria on the Isola del Giglio, a beautiful island off the coast of Tuscany. And there we squeezed every last drop of fun from the rapidly dwindling days of freedom, gorging on proper pizzas, sun-bathing and leaping from rocky promontories into the warm and sparkling Mediterranean. The post-finals week was the last of a series of short-but-intense expeditions that had punctuated the last couple of years of my undergraduate life. By then, I'd stopped being a reluctant medical student and, as the number of slow-burning friendships multiplied, I revelled in a tight comradeship born of enduring umpteen gruelling examinations. There was also a mounting exhilaration at the sheer range of medical practice and a waking up to the immense importance of healthcare.

Then, the real grind began, with my first job. I was relieved that I'd anticipated the monastic existence doctors were said to lead in their early postgraduate years by investing so much of my undergraduate time in extracurricular activities. Certainly, when I started as a Surgical Intern in July 1982, in Wexford General Hospital, I quickly realised that I would need – and thankfully had – a serious stash of happy memories to keep me going. It was Professor O'Higgins who gave us ex-medical students our valedictory speech, in St Vincent's, and simultaneously welcomed us to our new lives as Interns, about to be despatched to various UCD hospitals. He exhorted all of us, in our first days on the wards, to get to know as many non-medical staff as possible. It would be they, he said, who would give us at least one encouraging greeting as we entered and left the institution. He also urged us to recognise that most of what we needed to learn in that challenging first year could be learned from the nurses we'd meet, in every corner of our new hospital. I needed no convincing of this. I was always happy to have a friendly nurse by my side, in everything I did as a young medic.

Professor O'Higgins' advice was a tad surprising, but invaluable. And if I got anything right as an Intern, it was mainly by following his tips. First, by realising that a smile or a wave from the porter, security man or cleaner can actually make your day, whether you're coming or going. So, from my very first week as a doctor, I sought the name of every staff member I met. Second, it was from the friendly nurses in the operating theatre, who I first met on a whirlwind introductory tour of the hospital, and from the formidable sister running the men's surgical ward, that I learned most of what I needed to practise basic medicine for the next six months. And much more besides. I don't know if it was fate, but after a preliminary visit to Wexford General, I travelled home to Dublin to hang out with my old school friends for the weekend. As it happened, they'd decided to head to the Strawberry Fair in Enniscorthy, County Wexford, on the Saturday. Having spent the latter part of the day roaming the busy town, we ended up in a packed Antique Tavern, where I bumped into the very team of medics and nurses that I was due to join in Wexford that Monday. And such was the fun they were clearly having, and such was their wonderful friendliness, that I readily accepted an invitation to go back with them to Wexford, for a party. The Dublin gang headed home shortly afterwards, and I wandered off with the new friends I'd just met. It marked the start of a fast and furious first year in hospital medicine.

One of the perennial complaints of medical graduates in these islands is that they're not properly prepared by medical school for the reality of life on the hospital ward, never mind the emergency department, operating theatre or outpatient clinic. I certainly get this point of view, although almost four decades after my own first day as an Intern, I'm still not sure that a truly comprehensive preparation is possible. In my case, I was well used to hard physical and mental work, and I was accustomed to studying (or partying) until the early hours. I'd spent time in Monaghan General Hospital, which was comparable to Wexford, so I had some sense of how a county hospital worked. I was especially blessed in having spent time with inspiring surgeons in Zambia and Dublin. And there was no doubt that my hands-on experience in Monze was crucial to handling what the Intern year threw at me.

Still, nothing could have equipped me fully for the simple, hard fact that one day I was a (relatively care-free) medical student, and the next I was an *actual* doctor, carrying an enormous weight of expectation and responsibility. In truth, little beyond deliberate torture with sleep deprivation could have made me ready for the vast number of hours I was rostered to work from the first week. And no mere words could have consoled me when I learned that I wouldn't get to see the Rolling Stones play to 70,000 fans in Slane on a beautiful sunny Sunday at the end of that July. Or that my last festival for 40 years would be the Bob Marley gig in Dalymount Park, back in 1980.

For the next year, indeed for much of the next three years, I worked a one-in-two roster, so I was on duty every other night of the week and every second weekend. In practice, this meant that I would get out of bed in the doctors' residence (the Res) at about 7.00 a.m., grab a quick breakfast of tea and toast in the canteen, head to the operating theatre for instructions, undertake a hurried scouting review of all 'my' inpatients, then accompany the team on a formal ward round, after which I began the morning tasks. This meant taking umpteen blood samples from patients, labelling and sending them off, phoning the laboratory, visiting the radiology department for reports, ringing other hospitals for information or to arrange referrals, and fielding calls from GPs about patients they wanted to refer urgently, or who'd been discharged recently and now had problems. After a hurried lunch, the afternoon jobs had to be done. This often meant I had to 'clerk' up to twenty new patients who needed admission. I had to systematically record their presenting complaints, relevant medical back stories and initial diagnostic findings at the bedside, before the senior team members reviewed their case.

The days were always busy and, even if I was off that night, I wouldn't finish until about 7.00 p.m. If I was on, I might find myself assisting in theatre until late in the evening, gradually undertaking more and more minor surgery, like abscess drainage, appendicectomy or basic orthopaedic procedures, under close supervision by senior team members. And, almost invariably, the emergency list would start at about teatime and go on for hours. So I mightn't get back to my room until 10.00 or 11.00 p.m., after a final routine review of the inpatients and finishing outstanding jobs. Even after I'd gotten to bed, I was highly likely to be called back to the wards for minor issues, like prescribing pain medication or checking post-operative patients with a fever or oozing wound. By 7.00 a.m. on Tuesday, if I was unlucky, I might only have had two or three consecutive hours' sleep. And then the day began again, a little less draining for knowing that I would probably get back to the Res by 7.00 p.m. After that, the night was mine, to relax, or to start studying for the postgraduate exams.

Intern life was exhilarating, exhausting and sometimes frightening. What made it bearable was that most of the people I met were cheerful and fair-minded. There was the formidable ward sister who flung the windows wide open every morning in Male Surgical, to let the freezing fresh air in, long before ventilation science described the benefits of such practices.

There were the good-humoured and brilliant junior surgeons in the team, Raj Dhumale and Stephen Sheehan, and two frankly heroic county surgeons, the consultants,

George Angus Lee and Johnny O'Sullivan, who operated every other day for as long as necessary and, in-between, held court in the operating suite tea-room. And there were the many good-natured Wexford people who staffed the reception, canteen, labs, portering office and mortuary. Best of all, though, were the lovely and mischievous staff nurses in the wards and theatre, who made life better than bearable. This might mean a night to remember on the sticky-floored discotheque of White's Hotel, dancing to Shalamar, Odyssey and Kid Creole, the summer's chart-toppers, or an occasional party hosted by a local plutocrat in the sort of big country house described by John Banville, but with added touches of *The Great Gatsby*. Mostly, though, it meant the simple pleasures of cheery chat in theatre or at the nurses' station, late-night water fights with huge syringes, or a terrible fright as you traversed the dark backyard to the Res at night, only for a spectre in a bedsheet to suddenly rear up in front of you.

Such antics sustained me, along with the intense new friendships, but gradually the job became very wearying and, like many of the graduates of the medical class of 1982, I regularly doubted my capacity to go on. I know that one or two did quit after a 'nervous breakdown', a euphemism for a psychotic episode, or needed psychological help for the bullying to which they were subjected by a couple of consultants. I was exceptionally fortunate in having such affable medical colleagues in my team, as well as two inspiring consultant bosses in Messrs Lee and O'Sullivan. Mr Lee, an alumnus of St Andrew's College in Dublin, was a former Royal Navy surgeon-lieutenant during the D-Day landings and, in what little time he took off, he was a sailor, gardener and angler. He was a joy to work for, combining a love of fun and good conversation with understated surgical excellence and dedication to the people of the county. The other half of the surgical duo was Mr 'Johnny' O'Sullivan, another superb surgeon, who grew up in Donnybrook, attended Belvedere and trained in St Vincent's before obtaining his surgical training in Liverpool. He was a gifted and devoted public servant too, and a hugely entertaining raconteur, whose spare time was given over to his faith and to music, as a singer in the Rowe Street church choir and Wexford Festival Singers.

As is so often the case in life, I knew nothing back then of the remarkably overlapping connections my career would go on to have with these two great men, but I rapidly warmed to both and was immensely appreciative of the start they'd given me in my medical career, and the opportunity to enhance my surgical skills. This included moving on from my rather basic lessons in Zambia to a sort of solo appendicectomy: neatly opening an abdominal wall above the right groin with a scalpel, popping in a gloved finger to locate and then tie-off a gangrenous appendix, before removing it, and inserting some neat stitches afterwards. First steps, but essential, and quietly exciting, especially with the gorgeous theatre nurse batting her eyelids at you, approvingly.

I wasn't so grateful to the Department of Health, however, and as with generations of Irish medical graduates, I found myself drifting into almost irretrievable cynicism after learning that the reason I was permanently and utterly exhausted was almost entirely financial. In short, once I'd worked my basic 40 hours in a week in Wexford, the subsequent hours were paid at about 88 per cent of the basic hourly rate; above 60 hours, the rate fell to about 50 per cent of the normal rate. So, the more hours I worked, the less I – and all my non-consultant colleagues – got paid. And the less medical manpower cost the state. Professor Pat Plunkett, a former consultant colleague in St James' Hospital in Dublin, did some calculations 20 years ago in the *Irish Times*, and he reckoned that in the 1980s and 1990s, it cost the Department of Health about 1.3 times 'the basic medical salary' to get 2.5 times 'the basic medical hours', because the typical Intern worked an *average* of 104 hours per week. So, employing just one Irish medical trainee saved them the expense and bother of employing or training one more to staff the country's health service. 'Two for the price of one,' we called it. This generation talks of 'Yellow Pack' doctors.

The problem for the presumably gleeful civil servants is that this sowed the seeds of the current medical manpower crisis, the hostility between so many doctors-in-training and the department, and the 700-plus consultant vacancies in Irish hospitals. The thing that policymakers just did not get – and still don't seem to get – is that *too long a sacrifice makes a stone of the heart*. They have created a terrible but understandable and enduring cynicism among medics. In practice, this meant that when I was an Intern in Wexford, I frequently found myself on the brink of prescribing the wrong drug dose, snipping the wrong vessel in the bloody depths of an open abdomen, or mistaking *angor animi* – the often-reliable terror of impending death in a cardiac patient – for mere anxiety. Sometimes, at 3.00 in the morning, I'd be able to shake off the fatigue-induced brain fog with a coffee. Or, if I was lucky, a kindly nurse might double-check that 'we' were doing the right thing. The fatigue meant tasks took three times longer to do after I'd been up for most of the previous 72 hours, and it brought a perpetual fear in its wake. A fear of making a terrible mistake, the sort I read about often in the press and in the case reports of the Medical Protection Society, the medics' insurance body. Alas, a constant fear can ferment and turn to anger.

There was also resentment because most Interns, like me, had student bank loans to pay off, so we knew that the longer we worked for the state, the less likely we were to have a car to drive home, or a sun holiday to look forward to. And in those days, exams and courses were not subsidised, even though they were indispensable if you wished to progress in your career. Not surprisingly, most of my wages were gone once I'd repaid my loan instalment, bought some medical textbooks, or paid for a return train journey to Dublin to visit my mother. In reality, my way of dealing with that was to postpone the resentment and focus on the clinical work, of which there was plenty. There were so many absorbing or worrying cases that it was as much as I could do to put in the hours and read the literature afterwards. Most of the issues related to the surgery being done in the operating theatre, so surgical techniques, pathology, basic anaesthesia and pre-op preparation were at the top of my reading list. And most of the challenges were to do with the sheer volume of tests to do, and results to pursue, and getting them done in time to get the patient to theatre.

Nonetheless, there were occasions when I thought, *What in God's name am I doing here?* Like the time, within days of my arrival, an unfortunate man on the surgical ward died as a result of blood loss from a vessel that had been eroded by a tumour which we couldn't stop and couldn't replace fast enough. That was a frightening episode: for the poor patient, obviously, but also for this young Intern and the nursing staff who looked on distraught as the man succumbed, despite the heroic efforts of everyone available in the hospital that night. That was yet another scenario that I read up on afterwards and have dreaded ever since.

As part of my training, I also had to attend the 'Casualty Department' periodically. I have never forgotten one of my very first such cases. I'll call him Joe. He was a gentle, homeless old man with mental health issues, who lived in a person-shaped sleeping bag made from the kind of waterproof clothes usually worn by trawlermen. He mostly slept under hedges or on benches and rarely took off his oilskins or wellington boots, so when he arrived one evening in need of attention and we removed his kit, the miasma that emanated from his macerated, maggot-infested lower limbs was enough to empty the department for an hour. This poor abandoned soul was the first of countless similar individuals I got to know in my subsequent career. And once the fumes had evaporated, it was the tender mercy of the nurse looking after her patient that stayed with me. I was haunted for years afterwards by Joe's extreme gratitude for the tea and sandwiches she brought him, as his feet soaked in a bucket of pink potassium permanganate.

Those six months in Wexford were surprising, shattering and inspiring, in turn, but like so much of the early part of my medical career, they passed in a haze of fatigue and brain strain. And then, for me, it was back to St Vincent's in Dublin for another six months as a Cardiology and Neurology Intern. This meant that I worked for three months with Dr Brian Maurer, a hugely vivacious cardiologist, and two suitably cerebral consultant neurologists at the hospital, Dr Eddie Martin and Dr Michael Hutchinson. Again, I was on a one-in-two, but this time I was working in a huge multistorey building, which was run like a well-oiled machine by the Sisters of Charity. We live now in a highly secularised country, with an often-virulent distaste for the religious orders who used to be in charge of many of our hospitals. I try to avoid a rose-tinted view of the past, but the (sometimes severe) rigour of the nuns in 1983 meant that the building was always gleaming and the wards – run by nurses wearing starched bonnets and dazzling white uniforms – were spotless.

The consultants could be pretty rigorous, too. My abiding memory of Dr Maurer is of him roaring at me, in faux outrage, 'Luke, where the bloody hell are you when I need you?!', whenever I arrived late onto his ward round, typically after doing an errand he'd sent me on, like cycling to the Royal City of Dublin Hospital in Baggot Street to collect some cine-tapes from the angiography suite there, or rushing back from doing yet another urgent ECG stress test that was part of the job. Dr Maurer really was a character. Described as a *bon viveur* in his obituary, this passionate Clareman, with a German father, was brutally but magnificently candid. He once told me – grinning mischievously – that he used to smoke 'a lot more!' until he wound up having urgent coronary care during the latter part of his training as a cardiologist in the Hammersmith Hospital in London. He had a marvellous capacity to extract the maximum from trainees like myself. The fact was that he could be a hard taskmaster, but his charisma and direct style of leadership were just to my taste. I was exhilarated by the work in St Vincent's, even if it was never-ending and the boss was an irascible perfectionist. It was fun, too, joining him occasionally in Baggot Street hospital to assist at a coronary angiography. The subsequent multidisciplinary conferences with cardiac surgeons from the

Mater, like Maurice Neligan and David Luke, were a great introduction to inter-hospital cooperation across the city of Dublin involving exotic or complicated cardiac cases.

I always say that Brian Maurer played a pivotal role in my career, but in early 1983 he nearly ended it abruptly. And he taught me – painfully – the price of loyalty, the potential ambiguity of the word 'obedience' and the role of politics in absolutely every doctor's life.

Dr Maurer summoned me one Friday afternoon to say he was heading off for the weekend, but there was a special patient in the private hospital, behind the main building of St Vincent's, who he wanted me to monitor carefully while he was away. So we hurried across the bridge between the public and private facilities and paid a quick visit to the middle-aged male, who turned out to be a consultant colleague who'd had substantial surgery and was still quite unwell post-op. Dr Maurer introduced me to his friend, who murmured a few words of acknowledgement, and with that, we returned to the main hospital, Dr Maurer in good form at the prospect of his free weekend, and me ready to get stuck into the unfolding challenge of a weekend on-call. The following day, having concluded my routine chores, I again crossed the great divide between the two hospitals. This time it was with some trepidation, without the larger-than-life cardiologist at my side. The reason for my nervousness was simple. At the outset of our six-month tenure, the Interns had been told, in no uncertain terms, that we were not to go anywhere near the private hospital. It was, they said, completely outwith our remit. More than that, woe betide any Intern who transgressed in this respect, for reasons that seemed to be as much political as ethical. 'There be dragons' was about the only thing left out of the sermon.

To make matters worse, the special patient was unwell, so my cursory inspection morphed into an agonising dilemma. Eventually, I consulted the MIMS Therapeutics Guide, the pharmacological bible at every nurses' station in the land, and prescribed something I hoped would soothe the post-operative symptoms. Then, again rehearsing Dr Maurer's solicitous request that I keep an eye on him, I bade him farewell and hurried back to the main hospital. It must have been an hour or so later, as I was continuing my rounds of the public wards, that I got a bleep and rang the caller back.

'Hello?'

'Oh, hello, is that Dr Luke?'

'Yes. Can I help?'

'Yes, well, eh, Professor Fitzgerald has asked me to call you and get you to come back over here to the private hospital.'

'Oh. Is that MX?' I asked, hoping that it was the famously good-natured Professor of Medicine at the hospital, Muiris X Fitzgerald, known as MX, who was looking for me.

'No, it's actually Professor Oliver. Will I tell him you're on your way? He said you were to wait by the lifts.'

'Er, yes, please. I'll be straight over.'

My heart sank. It was Professor *Oliver* Fitzgerald, the same distinguished physician who had set out the stringent rule that Interns should *not* set foot in the private hospital, which seemed to be at least partly his fiefdom. He was at the tail end of an illustrious career at that stage, and an obituary later described him as 'forthright', with a 'stately air about him that could make him appear austere and aloof, [although] this manner belied a witty and charming disposition'. I hurried back across the bridge to the private hospital, not wishing to delay the venerable professor, noting as I did that the corridors and lift areas around the ward I'd not long before visited had fallen strangely silent, and all the staff normally to be seen bustling about had vanished. The doors to the ward were closed too until, several anxious minutes later, they opened abruptly and an exceptionally stately and aloof Professor Fitzgerald emerged, wearing an impeccably ironed white coat, buttoned all the way up as far as his college tie. His florid face instantly signalled the level of his annoyance, which seemed extreme. He then proceeded to pace up and down in front of me denouncing my insolence, disobedience and comprehensive delinquency in visiting the private hospital. Worse still, I had actually prescribed medication for a private patient, despite his edict to the Interns earlier in the year. His celebrated wit was nowhere to be discerned that afternoon.

I squirmed like a worm on a hook for the full ten minutes of the dressing-down, feeling genuinely fearful of the potential punishment. But I was also indignant. 'But, but … that's not fair!' was going around and around in my mind, although I wasn't going to add fuel to the flaming rage of the elderly academic. The professor kept shaking his head in theatrical disbelief and telling me that this was a matter he was 'minded to bring to the Medical Council's attention'. In the end, he waved me away with a look of pure disdain and said he would have to reflect on the appropriate sanction over the weekend and take up the matter with Dr Maurer on Monday. Not even the slightest protest on my part was entertained. So I slunk back to the public wards, my tail between my legs.

By the following evening, my transgression was the talk of the hospital. I was even more stressed than I had been for my Finals and, despite my on-call weekend exhaustion, I couldn't sleep with the prospect of being reported to the Medical

Council. This was something we all feared, although it was normally reserved for major sins of omission or commission. The idea that I might be court-martialled so soon into my embryonic career merely for following my boss's orders was a pretty appalling prospect.

In the end, I had worried unnecessarily, unaware of the nature of the medical politics that was at play between an elderly professor and a still-rising star of the medical world, yet to become one of the leading cardiologists of his generation.

I confessed my sin to Dr Maurer as soon as he started the ward round on Monday morning and he, in turn, wasted no time in seeking out Professor Oliver and giving him a piece of his mind. Rumour later had it that it was one of the most seismic clashes of that year between two of the hospital's consultants. And the consensus was that my boss had won. Happily for me, I heard no more about my misdemeanour, and it would be many years before I was again faced with the threat of a complaint to the Medical Council. If anything, the episode strengthened my relationship with Dr Maurer, who later took the opportunity to invite me and the other members of his team to dinner in his home in Booterstown, where he regaled us with drinks, jokes and anecdotes, and in return we all became his loyal fans for life.

Life as a Neurology Intern under Dr Martin and Dr Hutchinson was quite different. I was responsible for clerking patients referred from all over the country with odd, ominous or alarming presentations: fleeting visual loss, involuntary movements, abrupt unconsciousness, sporadic patchy numbness all over the body, headaches, burning facial pain or, worst of all, the creeping generalised weakness that heralded motor neurone disease. I had a decidedly ambivalent view of this part of my training. On the one hand, I found the whole subject of neurology enthralling, and at night I delved into mesmerising books about the pathology of the central and peripheral nervous systems, written by alumni of the world-famous 'Queen Square' National Hospital for Neurology and Neurosurgery in London. I was also entranced by the remarkable detective work of Dr Martin, a genteel older neurologist and author, and the youthful Dr Hutchinson, who was just beginning his stellar career and was as charismatic and telegenic as any of the TV medics I saw over the next few decades.

The best sort of detective work involved compiling a list of a patient's sometimes 'weird symptoms', like tingling and weakness starting in the legs and feet which spreads upwards to affect the upper limbs, face and bladder, intermittent double vision, night cramps, a rapid heart rate, fluctuating blood pressure, and difficulty in breathing. These would make absolutely no sense to me in the beginning, until Dr Martin gently elicited the patient's recent history and established that they had had a possible dose of gastroenteritis a month beforehand, and he would usually gently reassure the patient that the condition would probably settle of its own accord within a few months. It was only outside the patient's room that he would explain to the team that he suspected the patient had Guillain-Barré syndrome, a rare auto-immune disorder that can follow food poisoning, influenza and a range of other rare situations, including recent surgery. Who knew? Well, I certainly did after reading up on it carefully and seeing several cases.

And even then, I was impressed when Dr Hutchinson was able to divine a pattern in a patient with new left-sided blindness, uncontrollable vomiting and hiccups, and numbness and weakness in the arms. This turned out to be *neuromyelitis optica*, another rare, possibly auto-immune neurological condition that affects the optic nerves and upper spinal cord and that was wrongly thought to be related to multiple sclerosis in the early 1980s. My neurological diagnostic skills steadily improved the more such cases I saw, but I was particularly pleased with the progress I made with my newly acquired skill in lumbar puncture, or the spinal tap, which I was required to do almost daily as an Intern. This careful drilling at the base of the patient's spine was done to extract the glistening elixir that bathes the spinal cord and brain, which may offer many microscopic clues to disease. I even got to understand the basics of EEG maps, those records of the electrical brain waves elicited by placing electrodes all around the skull, which can help to confirm and categorise the many types of epilepsy, or to diagnose unusual conditions like encephalopathy or sleep disorders.

Sadly, the ward sometimes seemed full of the quietly suffering, for whom we could often offer little in the way of relief. There were high-dose steroids for the young mother with her new diagnosis of multiple sclerosis. There were a few effective anti-convulsants for young patients with intractable epilepsy. And there was the palliative care conversation with the middle-aged dad and his end-stage motor neurone disease. But, in truth, aside from the experimental options of plasmapheresis, or removal from the bloodstream of auto-immune antibodies causing diseases like Guillain-Barré syndrome or *myasthenia gravis* (another unusual neuromuscular disease causing weakness), or a whopping pre-emptive dose of steroids, there appeared to be strikingly few conditions for which there was anything other than a supportive or palliative remedy. I must admit that I was glad to reach the end of that stint. I had benefitted immensely from the wisdom of the two brilliant neurologists, and their remarkable ability to spot a pattern amid a welter of bizarre symptoms and signs, but, aside from the fascinating diagnostic process, neurology in the early 1980s seemed often to lead to a therapeutic cul de sac.

And yet, for the rest of my career I deployed the experience I acquired over those three months, and I have watched in fascination as neurological research and innovation have transformed the diagnosis and treatment of diseases of the central and peripheral nervous system. Frankly, I suspect that if I were an Intern today, I might well settle on neurology as a career.

It is said that finding your tribe can be transformational, and that is what I discovered at the end of my twelve months as an Intern, when, thanks to a glowing reference from Dr Maurer, I found a job as a fully-fledged senior house officer (SHO) in the A&E department at St James's Hospital in Dublin. This was situated at one end of the South Circular Road, in the grounds of a former workhouse and foundling hospital. Locally known as St Kevin's (the old post-civil war name) or as The Union (Workhouse), the hospital was actually a collection of buildings with different functions on a then gloomy campus surrounded by public housing projects. The most famous of these – or infamous, as it became – was Fatima Mansions in Rialto, along the southern boundary of the hospital.

The A&E department was based in a block near the South Circular Road gate and was a compact affair. The walking entrance was on the city-centre side of the block and in the days before Triage, which is the formal assessment of clinical urgency, an SHO like me would spend part of the day in one room just inside the entrance, looking after the 'walking wounded', with their facial lacerations, broken limbs or head injuries. The treatment of these was undertaken in an adjacent room, but periodically I would be brought out of the front room to visit the busy part of the department, in the back, where the patients were all lined up on trolleys and were often extremely ill. A nurse would take me round to each patient and point out the various issues and problems they needed me to sort. But the real glory of the department in 1983 was that the nurses were so well-versed and experienced that they presented most of the cases in an easily digested package for a young doctor to manage. They took a preliminary medical history from the patient on their arrival, came up with a provisional working diagnosis, took bloods and inserted an IV line, and called the doctor only when an actual medical decision or intervention was required. And they, the nurses, were ready for the doctor to make that decision or that phone call.

I loved the department at St James: the busyness, the cut-and-thrust, and the whole sense of doing something useful. And I loved the nurses, their boundless good cheer, magnificent competence and can-do attitude. I enjoyed learning how to stitch lacerations at speed, and neatly, how to apply moderately tidy plaster-of-Paris, and how to deal quickly and calmly with the conveyor belt of cases. There was a delightful synergy between the medical and nursing staff, an often-wordless communication that had people working together efficiently, based on mutual respect, experience and trust.

That isn't to say that it was always a frictionless joy. The job was just as tiring as my Internship, and the only time for a chat was usually over a hasty cup of 'Irish hospital coffee' in the staff room (actually a sort of fake coffee involving chicory and apparently homeopathic amounts of real coffee). There, as often as not, you'd find a member of An Garda Síochána motorcycle corps, an honorary member of the department crew, having his break with the nurses, myself and Stan O'Leary, the department's Registrar and de facto leader. The caseload reflected the grinding lives of so many people in the Liberties area of Dublin in the early 1980s. There was all the tobacco stuff, with heart, lung and blood vessel disease and stroke, the complications of chronic alcohol consumption, with accidents, assaults, gastritis, brain and liver failure and – reflecting unemployment levels of up to 60 per cent in the area around the hospital – the bitter fruits of pure poverty: overcrowding, domestic violence, and despair.

Then there was heroin. In the late 1970s, with the Russian invasion of Afghanistan and the Iranian Revolution, a tsunami of the drug flooded Europe as traditional policing structures in those countries collapsed and poppy farming, the source of the opiate, flourished. Legend has it that Larry Dunne, the organised crime boss, and his family (themselves from the Liberties), spotted an opportunity and began to import heroin from London, Paris and Amsterdam into Dublin, often through Dún Laoghaire. By the early 1980s, thousands of young people in the inner city, and around St James', were addicted to heroin, sometimes smoked ('chasing the dragon' as it was called), but mostly injected. A few middle-class youngsters also got involved as some of the drugs were diverted locally from the Dún Laoghaire mailboat, and a few young people I knew in the Borough died, but the numbers of victims in the county were minimal compared with the misery, medical mayhem and mortality due to heroin consumption in the city centre. This was particularly the case in Fatima Mansions, which was gradually being vacated by its older residents, who were replaced by a much more transient and antisocial population.

I was largely unaware of the bigger picture in the inner city at that time, but I quickly became intimately acquainted with the actual victims. Almost always young men, they arrived regularly through the ambulance entrance at the back of the department, unrousable, with the giveaway 'pinpoint' pupils, turning a dark shade of blue. This indicated that the brain's breathing reflex had been 'turned off' by smoked or injected heroin or oral methadone, a heroin substitute prescribed back then at the Jervis Street drug clinic, and that the levels of oxygen in the bloodstream were falling to lethal levels. (Brain death is traditionally said to occur after three to five minutes of oxygen deprivation.)

It is thought that opioids fit into specific brain receptors that drive breathing and basically switch them off, although adding other 'downer' drugs, like alcohol or benzodiazepine sleeping medications, will accelerate and exacerbate the risk of death. Sometimes users will die with a needle in their arms, but mostly the overdose occurs over minutes or even hours. I was also introduced to the 'lab rat' aspect of opiate addiction, which I never forgot. In short, once the antidote, naloxone, also known as Narcan, was injected into their veins, many of these heroin overdose victims would wake up suddenly and violently. They would often become very agitated and abusive, accusing the staff of 'wrecking (their) buzz' before ripping out their intravenous lines and angrily exiting the department, spraying the Resus Room and doors with bloody saline as they went.

Their behaviour, as I learned, was driven almost entirely by an unthinking, or 'brainstem', craving. And really, the key to understanding what happens when people use certain drugs, like opiates, cocaine, alcohol or benzodiazepines, is that, beyond a certain threshold of use (in other words, measured by time *and* quantity), free or rational thinking stops, and people begin to behave impulsively, driven by appetites that are below the brain's thinking cortex and in the primordial part of the brain, or limbic system. This underpins everyone's moods, and when it is damaged or poisoned, it can make people dramatically fearless, aggressive or hypersexual.

I suspect that the lack of gratitude for their lives being saved was the thing that first shocked every young nurse and doctor starting out in the A&E department at St James' in those days, but this was soon replaced by indignation when the same victim was found robbing the staff lockers a few days later. Or by alarm, when he was brought back to the department by ambulance not long after his first visit, in the same inert state as before, and sometimes died. That was when we began to appreciate that the half-life, or duration of effect, of the antidote was fatally shorter than the half-life of the original poison, the injected or swallowed opiate. In other words, the duration of action of an opiate like heroin, morphine or methadone can be measured in many hours or days, whereas the naloxone effect may wear off after 45 minutes.

The solution was relatively simple, and it is one I recommend to this day. The naloxone needed to be given into the muscle of the thigh to provide a slow-release or 'depot' effect, which would carry the victim through the relapse that may otherwise happen a half-hour or so after they'd bounded out of the emergency department. The other advantage was that the victim does not wake up abruptly, but was revived gently, without the risk of acute angry withdrawal and fountains of blood. Back then, it was preferable to avoid bloodletting, if possible, particularly as the HIV epidemic was taking hold, and of course this was all long before PPE was routinely deployed in every emergency department. Another approach is to give a prolonged infusion of the naloxone or – nowadays, in the community – a nasal spray.

After six months at St James', I'd learned an enormous amount from the nursing staff, just as Professor O'Higgins had advocated. Mind you, I was exceptionally fortunate in working with a particularly inspiring group of nurses there at the time, including Val Small, Ireland's first Advanced Nurse Practitioner. I was also particularly lucky to work with Stan O'Leary, the lean, lofty and eternally upbeat Registrar in the St James' department. He had been an orthopaedic trainee and was highly skilled in that field but, for the sort of reasons I certainly understand, he'd decided to specialise in accident and emergency medicine. This was then a relatively new specialty, with the first Senior Registrar or higher specialty trainee appointed in the UK only in 1977. It was Stan, in fact, who explained all this to me as we sipped fake coffee one afternoon in the staff room. And it was he who suggested that Edinburgh, Derby or Leicester were places I could train, if I wanted to become a consultant in A&E medicine.

It was far from inevitable, in 1983, that I would choose a career in emergency medicine, but at least Stan had given me the notion of such a possibility. And the most useful thing he got me to do, indirectly, was to pursue jobs that were likely to be useful to me if I did end up working mainly in an emergency department. So I found myself working next in general and orthopaedic surgery in the regional hospital in Waterford, then known as Ardkeen. This was like a much bigger version of the hospital in Wexford, with more patients, more consultants and more options by way of recreation, be it in The Tower nightclub on the quay or trips to seafood restaurants in Dunmore East, with the usual gangs of medics and nurses. There was a substantial amount of emergency department work as part of the job, and again a group of very amiable staff who made life, both on duty and off, more agreeable than it should have been on a pretty intense rota.

After Waterford, with a little help from an unexpected quarter, Professor O'Donohoe, my Final Exams saviour, I was able to find work in the A&E department of Our Lady's Children's Hospital in Crumlin. This makes it sound like it was some kind of high-grade academic post in London or Boston, but the reality was that in the mid-1980s in Ireland, jobs, including medical jobs, were hard to come by. So I was grateful to get a post as SHO in Crumlin, even if it turned out to be as gruelling a job as I'd had to date. I still recall arriving in the emergency department before 8.00 a.m. on the first Sunday, in July 1984, and being 'welcomed' by the rather gruff Sister in charge. 'Throw your stuff in there,' she said curtly, referring to my rucksack and the tiny staff room in the minuscule emergency department, situated at the end of the hospital's main corridor nearest the front gate.

I did as I was told and in about one minute flat she had shown me around Dublin's premier paediatric A&E facility: two rooms, basically, front and back, with perhaps a toilet or two, a small desk in the centre of the main room where the Registrar would sit (sometimes reading the *Racing Times)*, and a packed waiting room. That was it, that was my induction, and then she said, 'I'll let you get on with it, now.' And that's what I did, as there was already a crowd waiting to be seen. I guess I'd seen several dozen paediatric cases by the following evening, which was my night off. You could call it a baptism of fire or learning the hard way. Either way, I was well and truly dropped in the deep end that Sunday morning. The following day I met the one other SHO in A&E, Mary, and the Registrar. Thereafter, Mary and I worked every second or third night and weekend, like a pair of robots. There was periodic assistance from colleagues in other specialities, particularly young orthopaedic SHOs, and the occasional visit from the 'bosses', Messrs Dowling and Regan. In those days, many A&E departments were run by consultant orthopaedic surgeons, who were largely 'absentee landlords', even if, like Mr Dowling in Crumlin, Mr Ward in St James and Mr Flynn in Waterford, they happened to be genial and supportive when you did meet them.

The main problem was that urgent healthcare is mostly medical, so while there were plenty of bent or broken bones to be straightened, the issues you had to deal with were mostly meningitis, viral rashes, accidental poisoning, abdominal pain, lung diseases, head injury or surface wounds. So, having an orthopaedic specialist as a boss wasn't terribly useful for preparing us or keeping us up to date with the many nuances of such conditions. That is why I learned most of my paediatrics that first week from *A Paediatric Vade-Mecum*, a brilliant old pocketbook originally written for the junior doctors in Birmingham Children's Hospital, which became my constant companion for the next six months. The rest I learned from the local grandmothers (who were not to be trifled with) and just from dealing with an endless stream of tearful or taciturn toddlers, infants, and bigger children in that order.

Several enduring themes emerged as I saw more and more children in Crumlin. First, most paediatric illnesses are self-limiting, and the level of crisis involved usually reflects the experience of the mother, or the experience of the grandmother (who often just 'knows' if a child is really sick). This means there are always two patients to be treated: the child and the grand/mother. Second, paediatric A&E departments can be deafening places, with the chorus of little humans in various degrees of distress, but the very last thing a doctor there wants to see is a child who is silent on arrival. The quiet, pale and floppy child is usually the sickest one, with meningitis or a severe brain injury, perhaps, so what is greatly preferable is the *noise-reassurance-remedy-recovery* scenario.

The classic is the child who bangs their head and sustains an egg-shaped haematoma, or swollen bruise, on the forehead, and is drowsy and gurning a little because the parents are anxious to not let her fall asleep. This, in turn, is because there is a remarkably tenacious urban myth that sleep in such circumstances is somehow disastrous. In reality, parents can usually be reassured if the bang was low energy (for instance, the toddler ran into a piece of furniture), and if the child is allowed to sleep for an hour or so, they will usually wake up and start bouncing around the A&E department again. No scan is needed because the front of the skull is particularly thick and seldom cracks without massive force, which is associated with much more obvious damage. And a scan *itself* can be dangerous due to the radiation involved, all of which has to be carefully explained to each new set of parents. The third theme is that the vast majority of children recover completely from minor illness or injury with sleep, a little fluid, and perhaps some paracetamol or ibuprofen. And the final theme is that they are then replaced by another child with almost exactly the same story.

One problem with absentee landlords was that we rarely saw the boss, and he rarely saw us or came to the department. I'm sure he wasn't aware of how overwhelmed we often were, or how exhausted, working so many hours a week with minimal pastoral or educational support. But it came to a head one day when both Mary and I rang in sick – a rare event for either of us, and I think we both may have had chest infections due to exhaustion. Whatever the cause of this unlucky coincidence, it caused consternation at the highest level in the hospital, the Board, and some days later we were summoned to appear before them to account for ourselves. I recall the gravity of the situation being impressed upon us by members of the Board, but I don't recall any great sympathy for our plight. I know that we were made to feel deeply inadequate for this failure to keep ploughing on regardless. Nonetheless, I believe that the fact that they had great difficulty keeping the emergency department open as a result of just two junior doctors being sick at the same time, meant that serious consideration was given afterwards to easing the burden on the department's medical staff, whose numbers were increased gradually over the following year or so.

The six months in Crumlin were not entirely fruitless or fun-free and, in addition to an enduring enthusiasm for paediatrics,

I managed to obtain my Diploma in Child Health (DCH). I was then lucky enough to get a job for twelve consecutive months in St Columcille's Hospital in Loughlinstown, in South County Dublin. This meant that I could move home with my mother in Stillorgan for a while, and out of the succession of doctors' residences and cheap-but-grubby flats and houses I'd lived in for the previous few years. I'd had plenty of fun and adventures, sharing accommodation with old friends and new, but by the beginning of 1985 I was becoming a little despondent with the endless struggle to find jobs, the seemingly limitless hours of clinical work and studying, and the general and personal economic difficulties of the time.

The small hospital in Loughlinstown was not far from Stillorgan and Dún Laoghaire, and I knew it had a slightly dubious reputation locally at the time, mainly because it seemed to have been run by locum doctors or visiting consultants. However, a job was a job, and the convenience to home trumped prestige. And, in the end, having a job for a whole year in one hospital turned out to be a real blessing in disguise. For a start, it eased the anxiety of job hunting, and I could focus on working, studying for the postgraduate exams I needed to climb the career ladder, and enjoying being back in my old stomping ground.

St Columcille's was euphemistically called Wicklow General or Bray District Hospital, and part of the pleasure of those twelve months was getting to know the locals, who insisted they were a breed apart from the Dubs. And they were. As was so often the case, the nursing staff in the emergency department and the wards were wonderfully friendly and supportive, and there was a real sense of community and comradeship within the small hospital. It was probably the first job I can truly say I enjoyed for the *full* twelve months, setting aside the pure excitement of St James'. In addition to the existing team in Loughlinstown, there was a radical development in the hospital itself at the start of 1985, when an entire cadre of new consultants in medicine, surgery and radiology were appointed simultaneously in order to effect a transformation of its running and its reputation. And in this, the new consultants, like my then boss, Dr John Fennell, a dynamic and jovial consultant physician, now Professor of Medicine in RCSI Bahrain, and Mr Declan Magee, subsequently President of the Royal College of Surgeons, were entirely successful. Observing this transformation as it occurred clearly proved to me that the reputation of a hospital hinges on effective medical and nursing leadership, which can be facilitated with just a modicum of managerial or ministerial vision. And oddly, to this day, I remember the very wise words on a poster on the main corridor of the hospital: *It's nice to be important, but it's more important to be nice.*

Another crucial lesson from that time was that the morale and mood of a group of employees depend very considerably on their leadership, and the new group of consultants really did spread hope and good humour everywhere they went within the institution. But sometimes there is nothing that can be done about external events. All the hospital staff were rocked by a violent event that left its mark on everyone. The murder, in November 1985, of one of the hospital's nurses, Maureen Stack, in her home in Sandycove, was utterly shocking, especially in 1980s Ireland when murder was so rare. I think the first we knew about it was when she failed to turn up for work on the cold winter's morning she was brutally beaten to death.

Her colleagues' normal concern about their punctilious colleague, friend and a young mother, turned to disbelief and horror as the news broke. That was the first time I'd experienced the sudden death of a relatively close colleague, but everyone in Loughlinstown was profoundly shaken by the contrast between the grotesque nature of the killing and Maureen's familiar good cheer and kindliness. The terrible fact is that the killers were never found, nor was a motive ever established. But it was one of those events in my early medical days that persuaded me that violence was as terrible a disease as any other.

In hindsight, I came to love the little hospital in Loughlinstown. It gave me an unexpected but vital opportunity to recover from the despondency brought on by the fatigue, self-doubt and insecurity fostered by years of exhausting shifts, debt and difficulties finding jobs. The relative stability provided by the twelve-month spell in one place, the kindness of the nursing staff and the regular doses of encouragement by young, enthusiastic and inspiring consultants were all transformative. I'd had time to think, to reflect, to study, to pass a couple of crucial exams and, by the end of 1985, three years after I'd qualified, I was beginning to comprehend what it took to make a career in medicine: stamina, determination, ambition and an enormous capacity for physical and mental work. What remained seemed to be a matter of luck and keeping an eye out for the right opportunities. By the middle of the 1980s, in my case, those opportunities clearly lay in emigration.

Brave Caledonia

By the end of 1985, the Irish economy and my career were both in the doldrums and I was ready to join the thousands of other young Irish people who had little choice but to emigrate. The only question was, where to? I briefly contemplated America and Australia, but they were both non-starters. The exams for the United States were seriously difficult at the time, and I had enough to be doing with studying for the local postgraduate exams with UCD and the Royal College of Physicians of Ireland. The expense of the US medics' entry test was also ruinous but, more than anything, I still harboured some old Nixon-era suspicion about the military-industrial capitalism that seemed to dominate American politics *and* healthcare. Australia was too far away, and it wasn't yet a routine destination for Northern Hemisphere medical trainees. For a while, like a few of my medical classmates, I toyed with invitations to work in places like Nova Scotia or Newfoundland, but really I was more inclined to move to the UK. Initially, I half-heartedly looked at jobs in Derby and Leicester, as suggested by

Stan O'Leary in St James', and by Bob McQuillan, St Vincent's first consultant in emergency medicine, but with no great enthusiasm or success.

So that's how I found myself in Scotland, at the end of 1985, being interviewed in the Royal Infirmary of Edinburgh (RIE) by Dr Keith Little, consultant in accident and emergency medicine, whose name I had first heard, reverentially, from Stan O'Leary. Dr Little was *the* man in A&E medicine in the UK, according to Stan, and Edinburgh was *the* place to train.

The RIE looked a bit like Dublin's Richmond Hospital, only replicated about five times and with pointier turrets. The immense Victorian sandstone building, with its imposing central clock tower, was a quarter-of-a-mile long and was described on its opening in 1879 as 'probably the best planned hospital in Britain'. Its pavilion layout, with huge balconies attached to all the wards, was inspired by Florence Nightingale's hygiene theories and its primary purpose was to maximise space between patients and provide as much ventilation as possible. Around that time, most deaths in the recent Crimean War (1853–1856) were thought to have been caused not by the soldiers' wounds but by a germ-laden 'miasma', or fetid atmosphere, in the military hospitals behind the lines. This prompted Nightingale, the legendary nurse-epidemiologist, to launch her crusade to improve sanitation in every hospital.

And this began with air quality. In later life, Nightingale went so far as to describe the Royal Infirmary as 'the best hospital in the United Kingdom' and she regularly referred overseas doctors and nurses there to see its layout and policies. I knew none of this at the time, but I thought the hospital was certainly the most spectacular I'd ever seen.

The details of the interview elude me now, but I do remember that Dr Little and the other interviewers were the politest medics I'd met at an interview anywhere until that day. I suspect that all they might recall of that first encounter was my Irish brogue. And I struggled somewhat with their Scottish burr. I do recollect that they emerged smiling from the interview room in the A&E department, and in short order offered me a post as SHO, starting the following February. I returned to my hotel near the city's magnificent Waverley railway station in a slight daze, not quite believing my luck, or that I was about to become an emigrant. Later that day, I celebrated by marching the length of the medieval Royal Mile, from the Castle at the top, to the Palace at the bottom, then north to the Georgian New Town and south to the University quarter. Everywhere, the architecture was exquisite or extraordinary, or both, and the buzz on the busy streets was spine-tingling. It all seemed almost too good to be true.

I may have broken one or two hearts when I left Dublin for Edinburgh at the end of January 1986, but, if my long-suffering mother was bereft, she didn't show it. She was quite stoical regarding my move, and pragmatic in her farewells. In truth, when I lay in my little bed at night in the shabby but affordable Lauriston Hotel, a stone's throw from the Royal Infirmary, in the days after I arrived, it was I who was heartsick for home.

Thankfully, the sheer novelty of my life as an A&E SHO in the Royal was all-absorbing, at least during the daytime, and I soon found myself swimming upstream in a torrent of new names, faces and practices. My immediate impression was that the department seemed to be a decade or two ahead of anything I'd encountered in the five Irish emergency departments in which I'd worked. For a start, there were three outstanding leaders constantly on-site during the weekdays: Dr Little, the first consultant in A&E medicine at the Infirmary, and the equally brilliant Dr Colin Robertson and Dr David Steedman, Senior Registrars, who were subsequently appointed as consultants in the department. There was also a handful of energetic Registrars (mid-level trainees), and about a dozen SHOs, or first- and second-year doctors.

There were over 40 nursing staff under the direction of the demure but steely Sister Hazel Davidson, an Irish woman, plus a considerable number of porters, care assistants, cleaners, plaster technicians and dedicated secretaries. Another way of putting it is that there seemed to be almost as many people staffing the A&E department at the city end of the RIE as worked in the whole of Loughlinstown Hospital or in the surgical part of Wexford General Hospital. The scale of the department was just so much greater than its equivalents in Ireland. There was a large Resuscitation Room for the critically ill or severely injured, and this had its own x-ray machine to allow immediate imaging of patients. In my previous existence, a machine usually had to be wheeled into the A&E department to get a quick chest x-ray, if you were lucky, or the patient had to be taken down to a sometimes-distant separate radiology department, and often deteriorated en route.

There were separate areas for the 'sick' (Trolleys) and the 'walking wounded' (Exam). The Trolleys area was a space strategically opposite the Resus Room, with about fifteen cubicles for very sick patients, those with heart attacks, pneumonia, strokes or severe poisoning. This was where

Dr Little usually hovered, like a benevolent teacher on schoolyard duty, waiting to spring into action if a patient 'went off' or if an ambulance arrived with a case for Resus. Sometimes, he would head out in *Medic 1*, one of Britain's first 'flying squad' vehicles. This was a Ford Transit van, which, in between jobs, was parked outside the front door of the department, the monitors in the back plugged into a socket on the department's external wall.

At that time, Dr Little was already a renowned pioneer of pre-hospital medicine. This entailed getting skilled physicians to the scene of a crash, serious assault or collapse and starting critical or pre-emptive care within minutes, rather than waiting for the patient to get to the department, which might cause avoidable deterioration. Unquestionably, the *Medic 1* service, unique in Scotland, was the USP of the Royal and it attracted huge interest from the media and medics alike.

The Exam area had about fourteen cubicles, a large central space and a long counter where the doctors could do their writing, phone calls and x-ray inspections. And here was another real novelty: dictation. This was the first time I'd come across *typed* letters from the A&E department to patients' general practitioners. During the daytime, we'd dictate to machines on the counter. At night, we'd wander around to the little turret room where a real secretary, often the lovely, ever-smiling Liz Macdonald, would take dictation on the spot. This meant there was a typed record of every patient episode for all patients being admitted or referred to clinics, and typed letters were sent to GPs within a day or two of their attendance. This was a remarkable feat, one which many Irish and English hospitals struggle to emulate, even in 2021.

The staffing also included Clinical Assistants, or local GPs, who did regular shopfloor sessions in the department. They offered an invaluable combination of experience and a bridge to the community, which meant that there was much less friction between primary care and the hospital. There was a dedicated Dressings Nurse, who ran redressing clinics every weekday morning, and a couple of Plaster Rooms, with dedicated plaster technicians. One of them, the Back Theatre, as it was known, was equipped for minor surgical procedures and initial anaesthesia. Usually this entailed a 'Bier's block', which involved local anaesthetic being injected into the upper limb below a tight tourniquet. This enabled early manipulation of limb fractures by the more experienced A&E doctors, which meant that many patients could be temporarily sorted out, their bent wrists speedily straightened and plastered, and allowed home shortly afterwards, to be reviewed in the orthopaedic outpatient clinic. The alternative in many hospitals was admission for a day or two.

My first fortnight in the RIE was not just a professional rollercoaster ride but an emotional one. I'd arrived in Scotland with relatively little cash, mostly begged and borrowed, courtesy of the lean financial diet I'd endured for years in the Irish health service. So, although I was tremendously excited by the set-up of the A&E department and the prospect of working there, I was also profoundly stressed by the dwindling amount of cash I had left by the end of my second week, before I received my first NHS paycheck. And even though I'd reduced my expenditure to a bare minimum, living on a diet of baked potato and beans from the nearby *Spud-u-Like* café, I was down to my last few bob and destitution seemed to beckon. Thankfully, my prayers to St Anthony, or the equivalent Scottish patron saint of lost causes, were answered, and by the third Monday after I'd started another of the new SHOs in the department, a friendly Aussie, Rod, had invited me to share the garret flat he'd found in genteel Morningside, Edinburgh's answer to Rathgar, a mile-and-a-half from the hospital. This tiny, two-bedroomed flat was a godsend, even if we had to pass through the hall and climb two floors of the family home of the University's Professor of Celtic and Scottish Studies. The phone was downstairs, too, so there was a significant amount of shouting, 'There's a call for you!' Plus, the flat was so compact that you could hear every scrape of a flatmate's cereal bowl as you desperately tried to get some sleep after a night shift.

Still, I wasn't homeless. And even if I was homesick for most of that first six months, the main thing was that I could now focus on the other kind of bedding down. It probably took me a few weeks before I began to think that my new job at the RIE was like a dream come true.

The first time this occurred to me was in late February 1986, as the days began to lengthen and I was able to walk to work from the redbrick terraces and elegant sandstone mansions of Morningside, past the tenements, or multi-storied apartment buildings in Marchmont, across the broad sward of the Meadows, up Meadows Walk, past the Police Box (a.k.a. *Dr Who*'s TARDIS) and into the A&E department. The venerable Infirmary was a sight to behold as you approached it on foot through the Meadows. On the skyline to its left was Edinburgh's famous castle, one of the oldest and most besieged fortifications in Britain, and on the horizon to the right, about a mile away, the spectacular extinct volcano, Arthur's Seat.

So, according to the 'objectives' tick-box of this Irish medical emigrant, I was definitely making progress by my 27th birthday in March 1986. I had unquestionably found my tribe in A&E, as well as my new favourite city after Dublin. I had fitted in to the Scottish *modus operandi* without too much difficulty, beyond the language barrier. And I was thoroughly enjoying the work.

However, my domestic life was not so happy. Life in the shared garret flat was becoming a bit tiresome, as my Aussie friend had moved out and I was sharing with a new Irish GP trainee. He and I had different working arrangements, and I found it hard to sleep after the frequent night shifts with even a minimum of noise in the attic, or on the floor below us. I also began to have some of the strangest, most disturbing dreams that I'd experienced since my days as a small boy.

Twenty years previously, I used to have recurrent nightmares featuring a sense of drowning inside an orange lava lamp. Back then, I'd wake up screaming and nauseated. Now, I started to have the most intense and profoundly distressing dreams about my father, a bizarre development given that I'd scarcely given him a daytime thought since one or two incidents as a teenager, when his name had come up in conversation with rather insensitive adults (and I had just got up and walked away, to the bafflement of the grown-ups and my companions). But these new dreams seemed to emanate from my general homesickness, and they became a sort of lightning rod for the painful melancholia of the exile. It didn't help that phone conversations with my mother always ended up with her saying that she (still) couldn't 'remember' what my father was like, despite my ever-more-insistent questioning. This was to become a really serious issue over the following months and years, as I suspected a deliberate strategy on her part to avoid the subject, which was becoming a sort of obsession with me.

In any event, even if I was grappling with homesickness, settling in and the weird Freudian dreams, I threw myself into my work with gusto. This basically meant: work, sleep, eat, repeat. But there was always the Thursday nights out in the Cowgate pub, with dozens of other Irish medical emigres, post-night shift breakfasts in Stockbridge cafés, and exploring the Pentland Hills, just south of the city, with colleagues from the Royal. And slowly, almost imperceptibly, I began to feel accepted, and genuinely welcomed by my new comrades.

It was a bit odd initially, being the only Irish doctor in the department among so many Scottish and English staff, but I was fortunate in having had a path-finding predecessor, Tom Beattie, from Wicklow. He'd been a Registrar in the Royal in the early 1980s and had made an excellent impression with the senior medical staff and nurses in the department, before he'd found his particular calling (and a stellar career) in the paediatric branch of A&E medicine, just across the Meadows in the Royal Hospital for Sick Children, or 'Sick Chicks' as it was affectionately dubbed.

Then, bizarrely, in July 1986 a helicopter came to the rescue of my career. At least, that was how it seemed at the time. What actually happened was that a walker in Blackford Hill park, about two-and-a-half miles south of the hospital, fell and twisted his back. The hill in Blackford is a bit like Killiney Hill, but less challenging and, instead of an obelisk, it accommodates the Royal Observatory and an ancient hill fort near its summit. The parallel is important because there are gentle pathways leading from the car parks to the top of both public amenities. And they both involve a relatively easy stroll, especially in the context of Scottish outdoor life, where many medics (like Dr Robertson) spend their weekends 'bagging', or climbing, one of the 282 Munros, the precipitous mountains north of Edinburgh that are over 3,000 feet (914 m) high.

Anyway, when a phone call came to the A&E department at the RIE one afternoon to say there was a casualty on Blackford Hill with a back injury, *Medic 1* travelled to the scene, where the Registrar on board tasked an RAF helicopter to rescue the victim, who was subsequently transferred to the department with a minor back sprain. Given the relatively minor injury and the easy access to the hill by land, there was a hell of a backdraft about the costly call-out of the aircraft. In fact, so indignant were the senior staff that the poor Registrar was promptly relieved of her post. It was an ill wind, though, and I was summoned the day after the Blackford Hill incident to Dr Little's office, where he asked me if I would be prepared to take the post of Registrar with immediate effect. I was completely taken aback but, even as an insecure young migrant, I didn't hesitate to say, 'Yes, Dr Little, absolutely. I would be honoured!' And I *was*.

In most coming-of-age tales there is often an unexpected twist of fate that accelerates the growth of the protagonist towards adulthood. My appointment as a Registrar was such a moment. In truth, like many 'adult' males, I had until then been deferring maturity for as long as I could.

And while I didn't have a sudden epiphany, I did recognise a unique opportunity when I saw it, and I seized it. I didn't stop socialising with new friends in Edinburgh, but I did begin to envisage a professional future for myself. Before this, my career path was not much more than a kind of Brownian motion. Now I found, for the first time, that I was where I was *supposed* to be, in the Royal Infirmary, with ready access to advice and support, and a new-found ambition: the Fellowship in Accident and Emergency Medicine of the Royal College of Surgeons of Edinburgh. After that, a couple of years as a diligent shopfloor Registrar, followed by appointment as a Senior Registrar for a few more years. Add a little research, a certain number of medical publications and a decent number of presentations to groups of my peers. And then, well, a consultant post surely beckoned. Simple? Not necessarily, but it was now clearly worth pursuing.

My appointment as a Registrar fired me up like nothing before. Suddenly, I had responsibility for other staff, as well as for my patients. And three years after I was fully licensed to practise, I had had more than enough practice as a junior medical trainee. I had the benefits of almost four years in the Irish system, working all the hours, which was equivalent to about six years' experience in terms of forty-hour weeks. So by July 1986, when I was unexpectedly promoted, I was not just profoundly grateful for the opportunity that presented itself, I felt *ready*. For the first time, I appreciated the immense advantage of the previous years' toil in Ireland: it turned out that it was the perfect preparation for working in other countries' health systems. I joined a quartet of Registrars, on a separate rota from the SHOs, which meant taking charge of Resus Room cases, so the workload immediately became more complex and more demanding. It became more interesting, too, as the gravity of the cases was usually more severe than what was going on in Exam. Although not always, of course. I do remember the odd case that turned out to be less dramatic than the initial advance radio call would suggest.

The Blackford helicopter case was one example, but there was also the motorcyclist who had come off his 1000cc bike at speed and spun about 50 yards along the road from the spot where his bike and a car had collided. The ambulance crew had properly assumed that there was a high likelihood of significant injury, visible or otherwise, and quickly immobilised the victim on a spinal stretcher, observing the usual precautions prior to taking him, without delay, to the RIE.

The forty-odd-year-old male was wheeled in on a trolley into Resus, where the team was assembled, this time with me in nominal charge, while Dr Little hovered nearby. As always, the staff went into action. The nurse started to cut off the immobilised patient's thick leather trousers to gain access to what was thought to be lower limb fractures, amongst other suspected injuries. Fortunately, the patient was fully conscious, albeit a bit sore, so I was standing by his right shoulder, facing him and reassuring him that he was in the right place and we were going to sort him out. That was when I noticed the sudden silence followed by some tittering behind me. In removing his leathers, the nurse had exposed the lower limbs that happily bore no obvious injury beyond some road burns, but she had also revealed a particularly expensive set of lacey ladies' underwear just above the very hairy legs.

In hindsight, the funny bit wasn't really the incongruity of the lace and leather combination in an aging biker (after all, he could have been a glam rocker in the 1970s, or an up-and-coming MTV video star). In fact, it was the look of utter disbelief on the face of Sister Davison that made us all roar laughing in the staffroom later. Following her initial shock, the rather prim and proper nursing Sister seemed to take it upon herself to replace the unfortunate biker's expensive leathers with the tattiest Bri-Nylon hand-me-downs she could find in the department's spare clothes cupboard.

Thankfully, there was always an opportunity for a laugh in the staffroom because the work was often pretty grim. Or if not grim, then serious. Tittering was unusual in Resus, as the staff often battled to prevent a fatal deterioration in a sick or severely injured patient, and not always successfully. Just reflecting on one run of cases, I think of an elderly man dying from a leaking abdominal aortic aneurysm (equivalent to a slow puncture); a motorcyclist who had crashed on the main ring road, leaving him with a corkscrewed leg, and his pillion passenger with paraplegia; a man cleaning windows three storeys up who fell to his death from massive multiple injuries; the teenaged horse-rider with a devastating head injury; and an emaciated patient clearly dying from AIDs.

What made the difference – and at the same time what was basically the same with each case – was the *drill*, knowing what to do after endless rehearsal, and clear instructions from the ever-calm boss watching nearby. And there was no doubt that we were all hugely reassured by the thought that the consultants *really* knew what they were doing. Mind you, the most enduring advice I received from Dr Little in my first year at the RIE was, 'Resuscitation is the art of organisation', which, almost 40 years on, it surely remains.

Later in 1986, I was successful in the examination for my Fellowship in Accident and Emergency Medicine. This was a genuinely significant forward leap as it was my ticket to upward progress into a higher specialist scheme, once I had the appropriate level of clinical experience and a CV with more than just a list of jobs on it. So I got properly stuck into the work, and I made sure I was in the department a lot more than the minimum. In addition, I started the somewhat nerve-racking process of producing my first few publications. I made progress with this, too, although I quickly realised that I was first and foremost a clinician, not an academic. A parallel discovery was that it's difficult to see a lot of patients and undertake the substantial amount of research, writing or committee work necessary to climb the greasy poles of medical or academic politics.

The other thing that impedes a career in research is a busy social life, which I continued to enjoy after the Fellowship exam was over. This included my new friends from the A&E department, but I was also in touch with home and over the year or so after my arrival in Edinburgh, I successfully encouraged my undergraduate mates, David Valentine and Declan Sheerin, to move over to Scotland, too. David actually joined me in the garret flat for a while, until he bought a flat on the southern edge of the Meadows, near Sick Chicks, and we moved into his spacious apartment with pleasure. It was just a short walk to the Royal and close to the university quarter of the city, but, best of all, it was situated above a proper Scottish 'chippy' where we could get hold of the Friday night staple: a haggis supper with brown sauce.

The couple of years that followed my move to Edinburgh flew by as I got into my stride. The workload at the RIE was immense but I was up for it and I was energised by the ceaseless learning. I was getting more and more adept at realigning fractures, applying slick plasters, inserting dainty stitchwork and all the other skills of the trade in Exam. In Resus, too, under the watchful eyes of the trio of senior doctors, I was becoming comfortable with a wide array of critical care, trauma cases and cardiac arrests, and I was fired up by even the smallest of wins. This could mean the successful defibrillation of a chest pain patient thought to be fainting but who had in fact developed ventricular fibrillation. This chaotic quivering of the heart – the commonest sort of cardiac arrest – was mostly fatal, unless you acted quickly, grabbed the nearest defibrillator and quickly delivered the right dose of stored energy, or shock, through a pair of paddles on the front of the chest wall. This was sometimes enough to stun the cardiac muscle into 'electrical silence'. And, hopefully, the heart's innate rhythm then took over again and, after the fuzz on the monitor screen subsided, its pumping action resumed and the patient came to, often oblivious of what had happened.

The profound satisfaction of seeing this happen was hard to beat, and it exemplified the 'quick fix' beloved of us A&E types. The other quiet pleasure at the RIE was knowing that we were at the forefront of resuscitation science and techniques, so it was here I first used what we called the Thumper, a mechanical device used to perform chest compressions and ventilate the lungs in cases of cardiac arrest, which meant that the team could actually think about *treatment*, instead of worrying about the effectiveness of the exhausting work involved in 'breathing and squeezing' for a patient whose heart had stopped. And it was also at the Royal Infirmary that I first used a MAST suit, or Military Anti-Shock Trousers, which was an inflatable device designed to close off the blood vessels of the lower limbs and the abdomen when there was massive haemorrhage: the thinking was that if half the blood was lost (internally or externally), it would be a good idea to turn off half the pipes in the circulation. We used to use the MAST suit for people with abdominal aortic aneurysms that had ruptured and, anecdotally at least, the younger staff in the RIE believed it sometimes worked, although it did fall out of favour in the early 21st century.

One of the major lessons I learned in Edinburgh is that *pattern recognition* is as important in emergency medicine as it is in neurology or any other specialty. A good example is the classic 'café coronary' case, which a good emergency physician or nurse should be able to anticipate from the ambulance call alone. This typically involves a businessman, having a few beers and steak with colleagues after work, who keeps talking as he forks the meat into his mouth. The lump of meat therefore slides into his open windpipe, or trachea, and he starts to choke quietly. Acutely embarrassed, he shuffles off to the Gents' where (a) he is found blue and dead five minutes later after his colleagues start wondering where he's gone, or (b) if he is very lucky, someone spots what is happening and performs the famous Heimlich manoeuvre on him, or (c) he is seen promptly in Resus or in the loo by an experienced A&E doctor, who quickly exposes his trachea with a laryngoscope and plucks the offending piece of prime beef from the top of the windpipe, with a curlew-like Magill forceps. I came across all three scenarios during the 1980s, and I still think that if people generally appreciated the 'typical' story, there would be significantly fewer tragedies in restaurant toilets.

And then there were the trips in *Medic 1*, our modified Ford Transit van, which had almost everything you'd expect to find in an intensive care unit, except a bed. The vehicle was despatched most days of the week, to locations far and wide, and the trips were often gratifyingly successful, even enjoyable. (If it was a long-distance journey, you might get a chance to try the various siren sounds or admire the rolling countryside outside Edinburgh as the driver described the local history.)

Not uncommonly, there were false alarms, and we were summoned periodically to the airport but were usually stood down by the time we got to the Maybury roundabout (the last one before the airport). Although once, we sped past and I thought, 'Yikes. This is for real!' But it wasn't. And sometimes we provided remarkably effective advanced care at home. I recall one case where we went out to a suburban house, where a young woman lay on the carpeted floor of the front room, apparently dead after a severe exacerbation of her asthma. And yet she was miraculously brought back to life by inflating her lungs with some anaesthetic gas.

We regularly got vital pain relief to distressed victims of accidents trapped in cars or building sites, and occasionally we got to out-of-hospital cardiac arrest cases in the nick of time. Others were not so lucky, however. And some expeditions were particularly disheartening, like the cardiac arrest case on the pavement of Edinburgh's Prince's Street, outside a Burger King outlet. This involved me and the team rushing to the scene of a collapse on the city's busiest thoroughfare and trying to perform advanced life support on the kerbside, as pedestrians stopped and stared or, more than once, stepped over the dying patient, despite our best efforts to seal the scene. It was only afterwards that I realised that this sort of thing probably happened in every thronged city in the world. But it still felt as if people thought we were performing in some kind of Fringe street theatre.

Sometimes, the expeditions were both disconcerting and dangerous. In the mid-1980s, the *Trainspotting* movie version of Edinburgh, seen through the eyes of impulsive and agitated drug addicts, was all too real to those of us working in the A&E department at the Royal Infirmary. I had had glimpses of this scene at home. However, the big difference between the heroin scene in St James' in Dublin in 1983 and the RIE in 1986 was that the addicts in Dublin lived and operated near the city centre. In Edinburgh, they tended to live in the most deprived parts of the city, situated as far away as possible from the middle-class, business and tourist areas of the city.

One such place was Muirhouse, on the northwest rim of the city, near the Forth. In the 1980s, Muirhouse was a lot like Ballymun in Dublin, except that the high-rise tower blocks in Edinburgh had better sea views. There was a huge amount of antisocial behaviour and violence, often drug-related, and a rising number of cases of AIDS. In fact, a heroic local GP in Muirhouse, Dr Roy Robertson, had undertaken basic epidemiological research among the heroin users in his area and in 1986 published a seminal scientific paper revealing that 51 per cent of 164 local heroin users who were tested, were positive for HIV infection. Even these shocking figures were thought by some to be an underestimate.

It was no wonder that in the late 1980s Edinburgh was known as 'the AIDS capital of Europe', because heroin was being sold for £5 a bag while, at the same time, the police had a particularly aggressive approach towards drug injecting. One result was that needles were being shared for months at a time in the city's many 'shooting galleries', the derelict buildings where wholesale drug-dealing and injection occurred. As the needles became blunt, they were sharpened on matchboxes until a fresh supply could be stolen from the Royal Infirmary or Western Hospital. At that time, the very idea of needle exchanges was rejected out of hand by the City Elders and the police.

I'd seen countless heroin users in St James' and in the RIE, sometimes with acute overdoses that required naloxone, sometimes with injection site abscesses or the first manifestations of AIDS.

But I hadn't seen any of them in their own homes, so I was intrigued late one winter's night to be called out in *Medic 1* to a 'collapse' in Muirhouse, believed to be due to a heroin overdose. I was perturbed to be told that we would need to travel in convoy with a police van, because the locals were prone to lobbing paving slabs off the roofs of the tower blocks on to the 'Polis' below.

It took less than ten minutes to get to the area through the evening traffic, with our sirens blaring, and the little convoy of ambulance, *Medic 1* and police van slid to an abrupt halt at the bottom of one of the high-rises. This was dimly lit by the few working bulbs in those streetlamps that hadn't been smashed, as was evidenced by the broken glass on the already littered tarmac. It was a freezing night and the area was quite deserted, which is probably why the policemen stayed in their cosy van. The ambulance was turned around for a quick getaway, as was the norm whenever we were called out, and the nurse and I grabbed our suitcases with resuscitation kit and sprinted to the open door of the maisonette, where our driver said the case was located.

We came through the entrance into a well-lit, warm and comfortably furnished home, which was not what I was expecting. The other odd thing was that there were two skinny young women sitting on the steps of a staircase immediately to the right as I ran in, drinking whisky out of large crystal glasses. One of them took a drag from her joint and exhaled towards me as she said, 'You're too late, sonny. She's in there.' She nodded towards the end of the hall, right in front of me. I was momentarily confused by this, but I headed on into the sitting room and there, beside an expensive-looking leather three-piece suite and a large colour television, lay a woman of about thirty-odd, in a flimsy dressing gown. To my dismay, she looked as if she was already on the verge of rigor mortis: grey faced, cold, inert, with 'fixed dilated pupils', the usual terms employed by medics back then to describe the key clinical features of death. She was also spectacularly thin, to the point of anorexia. The most remarkable thing, though, aside from the bruising about her arms suggestive of a heroin habit, was her open mouth, which seemed to be filled with foul-smelling pus. I shook her by the shoulders, as was standard practice, and said, 'Hello, hello! Can you hear me?' Unsurprisingly, there wasn't a flicker of life. I couldn't help feeling that she must have been desperately ill for days, if not longer. I was highly sceptical that she was even alive when the initial 999 call had been made. I made no further attempts at resuscitation and pronounced life extinct, or 'P.L.E.' in the forensic parlance of the time.

The nurse and I spoke briefly to agree that there was nothing further to be done, medically. It was as we shuffled back towards the door that I heard the screams of a baby upstairs. It was the dead woman's baby, as it turned out, as her friends on the staircase confirmed. This was the situation that the police and medical social workers had to sort out, after the *Medic 1* team had returned to the busy A&E department on the opposite side of the city. I've never forgotten that terrible case: the genuine indifference of the two women as they continued their partying, the pitiful plight of that baby, and the tragedy of its young mother, apparently one of my first 'Pre-AIDS' cases, as those fatalities involving intravenous drugs and bacterial infection were often called, before systematic autopsy and HIV testing began in the late 1980s. In this instance, it seemed likely that a florid pneumonia with lung abscesses had killed her.

I'd seen relatively few full-blown AIDS cases in those days, as we tended to admit them quickly through the A&E department into general medical or infectious disease wards. But, of course, by the second half of the 1980s the epidemic was in full swing on both sides of the Irish Sea. I think I only grasped how bad things were when I heard that my former friendly acquaintance from the Bailey, in Dublin, the gentle, good-humoured and self-deprecating Vincent ('Fab Vinny') Hanley, had died in Dublin in 1987 from complications of AIDS, at the age of just 33. Vincent, a native of Clonmel in County Tipperary, had gone from being a DJ on RTÉ radio (when I first knew him) to being one of the first video stars on MTV, in New York. Tragically, he became known posthumously mainly as Ireland's first 'gay celebrity victim' of the disease. But we'd all heard of less-well-known friends from Ireland who had succumbed to the disease from 1982 onwards, and who spent their last days in New York or London, out of sight and largely out of mind. This poor woman in Muirhouse, who personified the parallel HIV pandemic then exploding in the drug-using heterosexual populations of Edinburgh and Dublin, had done the same, well hidden from the rest of Scottish polite society.

In truth, by 1987, I'd already had more than enough of the heroin epidemics affecting Dublin and Edinburgh, and the thieving from the A&E staff lockers that occurred whenever heroin users were about, as well as the low-level, high-impact crimes like joyriding that brought crushed and crumpled youngsters through our doors, particularly at the weekends. And yet it was booze that was the big challenge. Even the party animal in me was coming to recognise that so much of our workload was the result of excessive doses of alcohol. I think that many younger staff in every A&E department could probably be called extremely sociable. It comes with the territory, I believe, a means of coping with facing the grimmest aspects of human existence, day after day, in industrial amounts.

But one of the other facts of life in an A&E department is that, the longer you spend there, the more your tolerance of the follies of youth – or, worse still, of old age – wears thin. I am reminded of Joan, a formidable senior radiographer in the RIE, who had spent more winters in the department than most of us in 1987, and who was well able for most of the tricky humans she met there.

One particularly busy evening, Joan found herself dealing with yet another incident of unpleasant 'interpersonal difficulty' between a couple who had been drunkenly squabbling, when the young male had lost his head and punched his girlfriend in the face. The young woman was being x-rayed by Joan that Friday evening. I think what irritated Joan most was witnessing another rerun of that routine feature of the night-time A&E department: the fighting couple making up after a tiff and smooching in the waiting room. So she was perhaps a little brusque when she asked 'lover-boy' to wait where he was while his girlfriend was taken into the x-ray room. The young man, having been sundered from the love of his life, was less than pleased with Joan, especially when she directed him, as forcefully as is required when dealing with a very intoxicated person, to sit down.

'Hey, who are you f—ing talking to, you old bitch!' he roared. 'I'm gonna report you to the hospital! What's your name?'

'Florence f—ing Nightingale,' came the instant retort from the radiographer.

'Well, Florence, I'm gonna make a serious complaint about you!'

Minutes later, x-rays completed, the young man was fast asleep beside his dozing girlfriend. An hour or two later, no major damage done, the young lovers were leaving. As he passed the radiographer's room, 'lover-boy' shouted out to Joan, 'Bye, and thank you, Florence!'

Needless to say, no complaints were received, but the 'Florence f—ing Nightingale' response went viral around the department.

Still, no amount of good humour or saintly patience could disguise the fact that we had a serious problem with alcohol-related presentations, and it must have been a crescendo of frustration that persuaded Dr Little to allow Melanie Reid, a journalist from the Scottish *Sunday Mail,* along with a photographer, to spend a weekend in the A&E department with us. Their vividly illustrated front- and centre-page report, published on 6 December 1987, started with the headline, 'Wild Scenes in Casualty … Night Ward Nightmare', and it showed a young man 'with head injuries, flailing around and refusing to cooperate' with the nursing staff, adding that the department was 'almost at breaking point coping with people like him'.

Ms Reid wrote: 'What we saw inspired and horrified us. Inspired – because we saw doctors and nursing staff who are simply a credit to the human race. Horrified – because night after night they deal with a tragic circus of senseless injury and assault – most of it stemming from drink.' There were three more pages of words and pictures, featuring a lot of blood, vomit and sawdust, as well as a couple of our nursing friends treating various casualties. I think this was the first newspaper piece I'd seen that so vividly depicted the reality of a night in the department.

I have no recollection of the impact on the staff at the time, although we may well have been momentarily bemused by the pictures and headlines. I certainly don't believe that the piece made much of a splash at the time. Nor did the more personal piece by Dr Little, who appeared on the front page of the *Edinburgh Evening News* on 18 August 1987 under a headline: 'Casualty Unit Grinding To A Halt'. He was very downbeat in his assessment of the capacity of the department to cope with the ever-rising numbers of patients at that time. His main concern was the cramped conditions in the old building and the lack of space to expand, combined with the morale of the staff, which was 'at an extremely low ebb', he said, due to the 'increasing danger of assaults on staff by drunken or drug-addicted patients'. His solution was to ask the central government to fund extra staff to cope with the 5 per cent annual increase in the number of patients, which already stood at about 70,000 attendances a year, and ultimately to build a new hospital. But he was well aware that, while the local Health Board wanted to help, it didn't have the resources to do so, nor would it until a completely new hospital was built somewhere else, or £2m was spent on a temporary A&E department on the old RIE campus. So downcast was Dr Little, in fact, that he was quoted as saying 'I do not see the department managing to exist in three or four years' time'.

It was a sign of his leadership skills, perhaps, that Dr Little never transmitted his anxiety to the medical or nursing staff at the time, even if we were all too aware of the difficulties of working in the A&E. It was no wonder that he was held in such high esteem (a piece of graffiti in the staff loo declared, 'KL walks on H_2O'). In fact, very few of us hadn't been threatened or assaulted, at one time or another and, by the time the latter article was published, this included my future wife, who had been thumped by a woman trying to rob from a store cupboard in Exam. I suppose that what was important in the long run, in terms of the newspaper coverage in 1987, was the fact that the situation was being recorded for posterity. The headlines would have been the subject of some vigorous debate in Council and Parliamentary Sub-committees, but medics are used to debate swirling around their work for years without any actual impact on the ground. After all, the habits of a lifetime *can* take a lifetime to change.

'What's for ye won't go by ye'

Achieving the Fellowship of a Royal College was crucial to my career progress but, even though I was immersed in my work, I was homesick and lonely. Happily, though, the end of my loneliness was already in prospect. In retrospect, it was only in late 1986, when my great friend from UCD, Hugh Comerford, visited Edinburgh with his wife, Sheila, that I realised I'd actually been working for months with 'the One', in the A&E department of the RIE. She had been on a week of night duty when I first arrived, so we only met a fortnight or so later, when I walked into the staff room at the back of the department one lunchtime. I was having my usual Cambozola or 'blue brie' on a chewy Italian roll, a speciality of Charlie McNair's deli, next to Doctors pub opposite the Infirmary, where many of the staff got their sandwiches. The very attractive but unfamiliar young blonde was sitting at the opposite end of the table, in her white nurse's uniform, tucking into her own lunch of salad or something else that looked a lot healthier than mine.

'Hello!' I said. 'Aimechrisimeonuvdenewdocterrs' (which was what she later told me she made of my unintelligible brogue).

'Oh, hi,' she replied. 'Hayyayyemhhvickeewuhkclee' (which was the first thing I heard Vicky Wilkie say in her Scots burr).

The fact was that neither of us could comprehend what the other was saying. She later said that I had a thick Irish accent, and my hearing couldn't keep up with her machine-gun patter. So we smiled and nodded politely at each other and finished our food in a slightly embarrassed silence, realising we spoke quite different versions of the same language.

But as we worked together, it was impossible to miss just how industrious this recently appointed staff nurse was, how kind towards her patients and how fun-loving. It was this same Nurse Wilkie who passed on so many hilarious stories about the department and its staff and the city. Gradually, as the months went by, I looked forward more and more to working with her on day shifts, and especially at night. This was because the department had usually been emptied by 2.00 a.m., and then there was time for a chat, and a therapeutic titter. And as always with Victoria Louise Wilkie, there were plenty of laughs.

One night she escaped to the staff room, almost bursting with glee after dealing with a 'lady of the night' in Exam. Breathlessly, she relayed how she'd been dressing the patient's hand wound in one of the cubicles, when she'd gently moved the large saddlebag on the ground beside her. This had suddenly and noisily started making 'a bid for freedom', she said, and it transpired that Nurse Wilkie's touch had switched on some of the equipment within. The patient had grabbed the bag immediately and turned it off without a word, but the silence had been deafening.

Initially, we didn't see much of each other socially, even though we'd become very friendly at work. In hindsight, our moment seems to have come about on the weekend of Hugh and Sheila's visit in the autumn of 1986, when we agreed to join a departmental staff outing to the River Tay, Scotland's mightiest river, where some whitewater canoeing had been arranged by one of our more adventurous comrades. Hugh, who is one of life's natural comics, was in fine fettle, as always, but Vicky hadn't met him before that day, so travelling north from Edinburgh in the back of the car, it was easy for Sheila and me to convince Nurse Wilkie that 'Nurse Sheila' was minding Hugh, who was on a *very special* trip with his own psychiatric nurse. This ruse kept us Irish amused for a good hour or so until we arrived on the banks of the Tay, where we were all allotted canoes and lifejackets.

This was when the extremely late night Hugh and I had had in the kitchen the previous evening seemed like less of a good idea. It wasn't that we weren't game, it was just that we were complete novices when it came to canoeing, and we were exhausted, even before we slipped into the one-man vessels in the calmest part of the river above the rapids. And we did listen moderately attentively as the group leader shouted clear instructions about paddling techniques, steering and what to do if we overturned. But there is no doubt that Hugh and I were being a little loud and silly, as usual, while Sheila and Vicky were being model students and carefully heeding the instructor's advice. Still, it seemed to me later, as we recovered, that the rapids had come, well, much too rapidly.

The whitewater began a few hundred yards from where we had set off. So it was only as we waited in the queue of canoeists beginning to drop down into a stretch of turbulent water, punctuated by large rocks, that Hugh and I realised we probably weren't quite ready for the descent. The next thing we both experienced was the sudden, shocking impact of the rocks against our helmeted heads, torsos and limbs as we were torpedoed from the upper to the lower reaches of the rapids, and then upturned, both of us. Sheila was also a casualty of the rocks, although she didn't seem to have been bashed about quite as much as us. She certainly complained less.

In truth, that was a scary half-minute or so, losing control of the canoes, being smashed against the sharp granite, then finding ourselves upside-down in the icy water. Happily, Nurse Wilkie, alone among us, had descended serenely and in an upright position. She swiftly paddled to our rescue and, without too much delay, helped us to reach the riverbank, where we slowly dried off, shivering, a little shook and very much more alert than we had been during our brief tuition earlier.

Years later, when he was my best man, Hugh recounted how my wife and I first fell in love 'over a cup of cold Tay'. In fact, Vicky and I only became an item some weeks later, in November 1986, after she invited me to a dinner party in her parents' home in Trinity, not far from the Forth river's edge. The company – our most entertaining friends from the A&E department – was perfect, as was the hostess's cooking. I confess I also fell in love with the apartment, which overlooked a delightful park and, like the libraries and bookshops of my youth, was filled with wonderful books and comfortable seats in which to read them. I don't think I ever felt so immediately at home in a new place. And the following day, we explored Edinburgh's magnificent Botanic Garden, nearby. I managed to get bitten on the finger by a cheeky young squirrel, and my new girlfriend and I were greatly amused when an elderly lady rushed over and urged me to get to the A&E department of the Royal Infirmary as quickly as I could for a tetanus shot.

After that weekend, in which I was truly smitten, Vicky and I became ever closer. We spent more time together, exploring the city, and discovering the pleasures of the more exotic ('Sloaney') New Town pubs, like Kay's Bar on Jamaica Street, trendy destinations like the Waterfront in Leith, or Whighams in the West End, for long, cosy tête-à-têtes over lunch on our days off, and our favourite late-night cellar bar, Madogs, on George Street. There, the soundtrack to our budding romance was provided by Level 42, Gwen Guthrie and Swing Out Sister. But at home, it was all Anita Baker and Luther Vandross.

And then, in early 1988, there was another unexpected but momentous development. I was offered an exchange post in Queensland, Australia, covering for a soon-to-be distinguished colleague, Dr Gerry Fitzgerald, who was a consultant in a moderate-sized emergency department in Ipswich General Hospital, about 25 miles from Brisbane. Dr Fitzgerald, a charming, kind and cheerful dynamo, is now Emeritus Professor in Brisbane and a former Chief of Health for the state, but in 1988 he was organising the 2nd International Conference in Emergency Medicine in Brisbane and undertaking major research into Triage. This was a pioneering piece of work that contributed to the development of emergency department sorting of people according to real medical 'need, not noisiness'.

Although Dr Fitzgerald would be much too modest to admit it, the Australasian Triage System he helped to develop went on to have a significant global impact, as it was emulated in the UK and Ireland and beyond over the following decade or two.

In truth, I desperately needed that working holiday, as it turned out to be. Even if I had never even heard of Ipswich, the compact antipodean city, I agreed to take over from David Steedman, my predecessor in the Edinburgh/Ipswich exchange programme. When I arrived there, I was genuinely amazed by the beautifully appointed and modern emergency department, which Dr Fitzgerald had largely commissioned for the hospital. Bright, cheerful and packed with all mod cons for resuscitation, trolley and ambulatory cases, and for Triage, it was easily a decade ahead of anything I'd seen in Scotland or Ireland, and it was a delight to work in. Vicky and I travelled together, and we stayed in the hospital medical residence, a separate terrace of comfortable little houses a short walk from the hospital. There we found ourselves living next to – who else? – a lovely couple from County Mayo, Mike and Jill Thornton, and their little offspring, who were the perfect neighbours for a pair of nervous newbies.

Gerry and his wife could not have been more welcoming, and indeed everyone we met in the hospital was extraordinarily kind to the new young couple from Edinburgh. We were promptly invited to barbeques and picnics, and even though the heat at one point reached 40 degrees Celsius, we acclimatized surprisingly quickly to the weather and the work. Of course, it helped that half the non-indigenous population of the area seemed to originate in Liverpool, Wales or Scotland, while half the doctors in nearby Brisbane seemed to be Irish. Again, the English spoken was a different dialect from our own – a 'stubby' was a small bottle of beer, 'arvo' was the afternoon, 'you beauty' meant good man, and so on – but we soon picked it up. Similarly, the lifestyle. Beers in the hospital bar after work, barbeques anytime, and 'Slip, Slop, Slap', referring to the tee-shirt, sun cream and hat everyone was urged to put on to prevent the remarkably common skin cancers that occurred on fair skin.

This was a good example of how the medicine Down Under differed from that in the Northern Hemisphere. The complications of intense sunshine, for a start, meant that one of the services provided by the emergency department (meaning by me and Gerry) was excision of worrying skin lesions. There were also the first signs of a serious obesity epidemic which, to Vicky and me, seemed hardly surprising given the number of people wandering along the main street in Ipswich clutching pork pies and Cornish pasties from the numerous pie shops.

And, despite the obvious affluence of the houses and lifestyles within the city limits, we were increasingly aware of the grinding poverty endured by the indigenous Aboriginal population, as they were admitted through the emergency department or visited by Vicky, who worked as a community 'Blue Nurse', visiting remote hamlets and houses in the bush in her little car.

There was also the really exotic stuff, like box jellyfish or Irukandji stings in sea swimmers, or bites from some of the deadliest reptiles in the world, including brown, black, taipan, death adder and sea snakes or – in the comfort of your own toilet – a bite from a redback or funnel-web spider or tarantula. In theory, there was no end to the hideous hazards of just leaving your home in Queensland but, in practice, as long as you minimised your time reading about them, there was a relatively small risk of such bites or stings, or even blows from larger animals, like kangaroos, hopping in front of your car on the highway. 'Tropical medicine', as such, mainly affected the far north of Queensland, with fearsome haemorrhagic viral diseases and so on. In practice, most of the stuff we saw, from cardiac arrests to diabetic crises, mirrored the caseload in Edinburgh and Dublin. The key difference, which remains to this day, was the far greater resourcing of the health service in Australia compared with that in the NHS and in Ireland. This meant that the medical facilities everywhere we visited (including in Brisbane) were bigger and better, and there were far more doctors and nurses than at home. It was in Ipswich Hospital that I first encountered a medic specialising in hospital administration. I often thought that that – at least *partially* – explained why the hospital seemed to be so well run, and to this day I believe that it is essential to have doctors – ideally with special training – routinely involved in hospital administration.

Vicky and I had a fantastic time in Australia. The hugely enjoyable trade fair, World Expo '88, was on in Brisbane, which was embarking on a metamorphosis from sleepy provincial capital into a high-rise global city. At weekends, if we weren't invited to a local barbeque, we travelled along the Queensland coast as far south as Byron Bay in New South Wales to spot whales, or up to Noosa, a blend of Malibu and Quinta do Lago. And at the end of our stay we took a campervan up north to Cairns, visiting rainforests, the Whitsunday Islands and the Barrier Reef en route. Snorkelling and exploring the still pristine coral ecosystem around Dunk Island was a highlight of that once-in-a lifetime month-long journey, although the 24-hour train ride back down the Queensland coast was pretty memorable, too. After that, we flew to Sydney to meet Jock Bone, Vicky's delightful great-uncle, a Glaswegian who'd been a 'ten-pound pom' in the 1950s, one of the many Brits encouraged to migrate to Australia and New Zealand after the Second World War on payment of £10.

Like most Irish or British visitors to Australia, I suspect, Vicky and I fell in love with the lifestyle. Frankly, with the conditions, the wages and the endless exotic extracurricular possibilities, it seemed irresistible. We deliberated long and hard over the question of a more permanent move. But the implications of such a relocation were painfully illustrated in 1988 when we missed the weddings of two of my closest friends. Having been my schoolfriend Peter Kenny's nervous best man at his wedding, in UCC's lovely Honan Chapel, in 1987, and thoroughly enjoyed an eventful wedding feast afterwards, it was a blow to miss the two Dublin nuptials, both with the potential for particularly mischief-making best man speeches. So, in the end, we agreed: an Australian future was not for us because we both really were family types and, in a crisis, home would be simply too far away. Thirty years on, having lost one cherished parent each, we are even more certain that we made the right decision.

Although Vicky and I got back to Scotland in time for Christmas 1988, it wasn't a particularly happy one. As she likes to remind me, I 'dumped' her unceremoniously as soon as we got back to Heathrow airport. The fact was that all those months living together, so up close and personal, had brought out my inner only child and I reverted to type by bolting, much as I had done for the ten years since I'd been ditched by my teen girlfriend. I freely admit that at that stage running for the hills had become a reflex on my part whenever I felt that someone was making plans for me.

Anyhow, I got back to work, more conscious than ever of the pressures in the congested A&E department at the RIE which, after the stint in Ipswich Hospital, looked distinctly antique and inadequate to its purpose. I was also beginning to think ahead and was planning to apply for a Senior Registrar post somewhere. I had quietly nurtured a hope that I might be appointed at the Royal Infirmary. Regardless of my extracurricular love life, I had fallen for Edinburgh and I dared to dream of climbing the career ladder at Lauriston Place, even with its structural deficiencies. I also loved being part of the growing team in the department. I enjoyed good relations with most of the medics in the building and looked not just to Dr Little but to Drs Robertson and Steedman as inspirational and peerless teachers.

I had begun to expand my CV, too, with further publications and a growing number of lectures in the Royal College in Edinburgh, and at scientific meetings in Edinburgh, Glasgow and Leicester. Perhaps it was the shock of the new, and my experience of the grinding poverty of the Aboriginal people and their consequent poor health, but I also began to see the world through a more political lens. I wearied of repairing the self-harm of so many patients that was almost entirely the consequence of drink, drugs or deep-seated pain. I continued to broaden my attention towards the social determinants of the emergency department workload – and on how so much of it was potentially preventable.

I think the archetypal case of this was a man who had been organising a fireworks display but, in the manner of so many fireworks mishaps, had gone back to reignite a particularly large rocket whose fuse paper had been lit but had seemingly gone out. In a matter of nanoseconds, I imagine, his life was shattered. As he bent down to look at the firework, the rocket ignited properly and struck his head with the force of a small mortar round, causing such anatomical devastation that the only thing my fellow Registrar, Malcolm, could recognise in trying to resuscitate the patient was the tongue, through which he drove a huge, curved surgical needle, with a thread the size of a shoelace that he then yanked upwards to keep the tongue from falling back into the airway. This saved the poor man's life, but most of his facial anatomy, including the eyes and frontal brain lobes, were so traumatised that I understand he never fully recovered. It takes a case like this, seeing it or managing it, to make you really appreciate that prevention is so important, so much easier and so much more successful than any amount of impressive or expensive surgery for trauma. I was certainly permanently persuaded.

I came across the lovely Scottish expression, 'What's for ye won't go by ye,' the week I started work in Edinburgh in 1986, and I began to apply it to any situation where formerly I might have said, '*Que sera sera*'. I initially thought of it as a kind of comment on destiny or fate. So it was a standard comment after a cardiac arrest that we didn't get back, or someone's failed job application, or a friend who was broken-hearted over lost love. Until suddenly, it applied to me. In 1989, another Registrar was appointed to the coveted Senior Registrar post at the RIE, and for a while I was crushed. I tried to work out where I'd gone wrong in delicate conversation with Drs Robertson and Steedman, but I never really found out. A theory I entertained for a while was that I had gone on one solo run too many.

The main example of this, as far as I knew, was the case of a man whose heart had been skilfully punctured by his wife with a single thrust of a kitchen knife (as the comedienne Jo Brand once observed, 'The best way to a man's heart isn't really through his stomach, it's through his ribcage, on the left'). I was the Registrar on the night he was rushed into Resus and being aware – in theory – that such cases had only one chance of getting out alive, I promptly opened him up, splitting his ribs and breastbone with the sharpest surgical instruments available, diving into the chest cavity beneath and sticking my gloved finger into the gaping wound in the heart wall, to plug the leak. At the same time, I got the senior nurse to call the duty chest surgeon and asked him to come to the A&E department as soon as possible.

Knowing he was on his way, I introduced a bladder catheter in through the hole in the heart and inflated its balloon to create a sort of tamponade, or plugging, effect within the ventricular chamber, which allowed the heart to resume its pumping action. I vaguely recall the noise and excitement in Resus at the time, along with my own beating heart, as the surgeon reached us within what seemed to be a matter of a few minutes. His opening gambit was, 'What have we here? Ah yes. I see…' He donned his gloves and inspected the gaping thorax. Then he said, 'The only thing I would add here, young man, is if you're going to make a hole in the chest, just make sure it's a big f—ing hole!' And he beamed as he went on to enlarge my tentative thoracotomy opening into a full 'clamshell' effect, with the anterior chest wall unzipped from side to side, like the maw of a moderate-sized shark. And that was it, really.

129

The rest was about getting the patient to the operating theatre and intensive care unit, where I learned later that he had not only survived but had been discharged. The only problem was that the following morning, I was taken aside by Dr Steedman for a quiet word, which turned out to be an unforgettable reproach, the gist of which was that Dr Little was, er, disappointed that I hadn't called him in, too. This was another case of, 'But ... but ... what about the laudable initiative and the success?' And who doesn't hate being a disappointment to their parent or much-esteemed boss? I had been so utterly focused on the job in hand and getting hold of the chest surgeon that it had completely slipped my mind to call my own boss. A simple error, maybe, but I still think it rankled with him, and I long suspected that it didn't play well when I subsequently went hunting for the Senior Registrar post. This felt like my own 'helicopter moment'. The truth, of course, is that the best man for the job got it. I was still profoundly disheartened, though, and I was reminded of the famous lamentation of Dick Tuck, on losing the ticket in a Californian election in 1962: 'The people have spoken. The bastards'.

And so, as I planned, sadly, to leave my adopted Scottish hometown for pastures new, I found myself checking the weekly vacancies page in the *British Medical Journal*, until eventually I found a potentially suitable job that seemed to tick most of the boxes: a large teaching hospital, attached to a university, in a big British city, near an airport, with a sea ferry and ease of access to Ireland. This rather unsentimental method was how I thought I selected the Royal Liverpool University Hospital as my next potential port of call. In reality, as it turned out, a subconscious bias was at work, and the connections with home would slowly become apparent over the following 30 years.

But there was one immense and incomparable consolation prize. My professional future might not be in Edinburgh, but as far as Vicky and I were concerned, there would be no more impulsive and immature only-child syndrome. In 1989, after a couple of months of separation, we were reunited. I grovelled. She forgave. And before I could change my mind, she accepted my proposal of marriage. If I had finally learned one important life lesson in in my time in Scotland, it was the most important one of all, which I should have learned in the previous two decades.

Love hurts. But not nearly as much as a life without love.

The Pool of Life

Despite what the more pessimistic might say, there are blessings associated with getting older. For instance, it took me over 30 years to understand why I came to love Liverpool, when it wasn't initially an obvious rival to Dublin or Edinburgh for my affection. But now it makes perfect sense.

My first visit to the Merseyside port was actually with my mother, in 1967, to see the remarkable new Catholic Metropolitan Cathedral which, in a backhanded compliment to the Irish, was quickly nicknamed 'Paddy's Wigwam'. However, aside from passing through the city in 1977 on the way to see Thin Lizzy at Reading, my next visit wasn't until 1989, when I successfully interviewed for the post of Senior Registrar in Accident and Emergency Medicine, the last stage of specialist medical training, at the Royal Liverpool University Hospital. This twelve-storey block of brutalist architecture, which the Scousers dubbed 'Fawlty Towers' due to its dodgy construction history, was situated on the edge of the university quarter, between Islington and Toxteth, a ten-minute walk from Lime Street railway station and a mile or so from the docks.

The city had much to offer me, particularly geographic and demographic proximity to Dublin, but looking back I think my fondness for the place was probably inspired by my admiration for six very particular men and their work. Inevitably, for someone of my generation, they included the motherless teens, John Lennon and Paul McCartney, the working-class hero Ringo Starr and the sweet-natured George Harrison. The Beatles may not have been 'bigger than Jesus' for me, but they were certainly the heroic geniuses of my musical youth. And the more I learned about them, the more I appreciated the affinity they had with Ireland and their many family and cultural connections with my homeland.

A much less obvious source of inspiration was Nikolaus Pevsner, the brilliant German architectural historian. Briefly interned in Merseyside after escaping Nazi Germany in the 1930s, he subsequently produced a magisterial series of books entitled *The Buildings of England*, in one of which I accidentally read about the wondrous architecture of Liverpool, which he said had more listed buildings than any other English city outside London. 'Who knew?' I remember thinking, absolutely intrigued.

And then there was Lawrence H. Jaffey, a tall, dark and handsome Brummie, who was a dead ringer for Magnum PI, with a hint of Jason King, from two favourite 1970s TV series. Lawrence, or 'the Jaffster' as he was affectionately known, had the requisite moustache, Savile Row tailoring and powder-blue Porsche parked outside the Royal. But even better than panache, my new consultant boss had wit and charisma in spades, which in one of the busiest emergency departments in Britain were indispensable. And, happily for me, Lawrence was exactly the mentor I needed.

The city itself seduced me, too. Historians think Liverpool originated in 1190, as a port for trade with Ireland and, unsurprisingly, a quarter of the population was originally said to be Irish-born. For a long time it was the 'second city' of the British Empire, immensely enriched by the wretched slave trade. But by the late 1800s it had become the New York of Europe, as millions of Europeans, including innumerable survivors of the Irish Famine, emigrated to the New World through the vast docks and iconic waterfront, a melange of Manhattan, Hamburg and Shanghai. This enormous influx of people meant that the city was one of the earliest truly multicultural cities in the world, with large and long-established Chinese, Caribbean and African populations, as well as representatives of every European nation.

The Second World War visited terrible devastation on Merseyside, as did the post-war collapse in manufacturing, and then dockside automation. By the time I arrived in October 1989, Liverpool was on its uppers. Unemployment in the city had reached 20 per cent or double the national average, heroin use was rampant, the Toxteth riots had left a legacy of seething resentment in large parts of the inner city, and the City Council – dominated by Derek Hatton's far-left Militant group – was facing bankruptcy. Just when it seemed things couldn't get worse, in April 1989 the Hillsborough Disaster in Sheffield saw 96 Liverpool fans crushed to death, through a combination of policing failures and flawed stadium design. The mood in the city in late 1989 was sombre, to say the least, and many Liverpudlians were grief-stricken.

The most visible aspect of the city's difficulties were the huge swathes of dereliction in the many parts of the metropolis flattened by the Luftwaffe during the war. And this included much of the area around Sefton General Hospital, in whose dingy doctors' residence I spent much of the first six months of my career in Liverpool. To make matters even more interesting, the window of my room looked out onto one of the great cemeteries of the city. So at night, I was often entertained by the sight of ne'er-do-wells scampering around the headstones and monuments as a police helicopter hovered above, shining its search beam hither and thither, and through my thin net curtain.

I didn't let this minor source of sleep disruption or the melancholic state of the great city get me down, though. I imagine this was because Vicky and I were engaged to be married in March 1990, and every telephone conversation with her was about the big day. I was also travelling up to Edinburgh whenever I had a free weekend to join in the excited planning.

And there is no doubt that, at the time, I really did have a rose-tinted view of the world around me, which included my new workplace at the Royal and the umpteen unfamiliar faces. Even as I moved around the city after work, thanks to Mr Pevsner, I ignored the dereliction and instead admired the many surviving magnificent buildings on the waterfront, the two great cathedrals and the hundreds of other listed buildings scattered along the river front and near the hospital. Or I searched keenly for echoes of the Fab Four's childhood, in inner-city terraces or the southside suburbs about Penny Lane and Menlove Avenue. The icing on the city's cake was the remarkable collection of Victorian parks, like Sefton,

Prince's and Calderstones, where you could spend hours cycling, walking or just sitting, admiring the ducks or other wildlife, including the locals.

The locals were a huge part of my love affair with Liverpool. It was the joking that first made me realise that Scousers were, more than anything else, a defiant bunch. Vulnerable perhaps, but defiant. Notwithstanding the fact that in my first week one of my patients at the Royal had told me to 'F— off back to Paddyland!', I quickly fell for the people of the city. They'd endured decades of disastrous downturn, and yet it was impossible to spend a shift, or engage in conversation, with Liverpudlian colleagues or patients without having a proper laugh. I reckon this Scouse stoicism – tittering in the face of adversity – derived from the difficulties faced by generations of people fleeing famine and persecution through the city, many of whom chose to stay. It is in that mix, I suspect, that the basis lies for my relationship with Liverpool. Human vulnerability, musicality, comedy, a vast cultural, sporting and historic hinterland with an enormous Irish input, and a defiance of the gods, governments and those who looked down their noses at their city. It turned out to be a pretty good match.

I often say that I gave my best ten years to Liverpool because I came of age there. Like most young consultants in emergency medicine, which is a particularly physical specialty, I was in my prime clinically, or at the bedside, during my thirties. The first two years as Senior Registrar in the Royal passed in a blur of marriage (a big, happy Scottish-Irish affair in Edinburgh), a blissful honeymoon in Venice and Tuscany, buying our first home (a dainty Victorian terraced house at one end of Orford Street, in Wavertree, with a pub at the other end auspiciously named The Edinburgh), and having our first baby, Ciara. By then I was in that zone of full-on commitment to my work, so after seeing her safely delivered in Oxford Street Maternity Hospital at 3.00 a.m., I turned up at the Royal to teach the SHOs at 8.00 a.m. That was how I approached work in those final days of training – with my then-trademark intensity – whether it was in adult or paediatric emergency medicine, plastic and burns surgery, gynaecology, neonatology, cardiorespiratory medicine, or a particularly inspiring toxicology stint with Guy's Hospital in London.

The final piece of my bespoke education was a Grand Tour of emergency departments in Belgium, Holland, France and Germany. I did this to see how they operated on the continent. The answer in a word? Differently! But it was a wonderful opportunity to appreciate just how much continental medicine varies between neighbouring countries, and how it differs from the Anglo-Irish model.

In October 1992, I was appointed as a consultant in the Royal. By this time, I had decided that my favourite clinical challenges were 'toddlers, trauma and toxicology'. This flowed from my time in Crumlin and Alder Hey, where I'd seen so many sick or injured little children bounce back gratifyingly after relatively simple treatment for their head injury, cracked wrist or asthma flare. It followed my experience in Edinburgh of treating so many seriously injured patients and realising that an urgent but systematic approach could often produce a calm and comfortable patient, cleaned, plastered, and splinted, lying on a bed and having a cup of tea within an hour or so. And it followed my exposure to vast amounts of heroin and other drug overdoses (Paracetamol and antidepressants were just as toxic) in Dublin, Edinburgh and Liverpool, as well as the inspiring teachers at the National Poisons Centre in London, who gave me a great enthusiasm for dealing with almost any poisoning case for the rest of my career.

Consultants must be much more than just good clinicians, so I was also particularly interested in education, prevention and communication – between everyone within the emergency department, but also between us and the world beyond its doors. It had become clear that the progress *we* in the emergency department were making in terms of the care we were providing wasn't always so obvious to either colleagues or citizens. I threw myself into this aspect of my work with gusto. And that really became the bigger picture theme of my time at the Royal. Real and exciting progress was being made, all around us and *by* us, and we needed to spread the message.

One of the best pieces of good news was the building of a huge new department at the Royal in 1994, which transformed the cramped old facility that existed when I first arrived into a two-storey, state-of-the-art department, with around 30 doctors, 100 nurses and 50 ancillary staff. Those numbers were just about sufficient to cope with our caseload of over 100,000 new patient attendances a year. These included about 200 cases of cardiac arrest, many critically injured patients, and up to twenty cases a day in our Short Stay Observation (or Obs) ward. This was an inpatient facility where we looked after patients with head injuries, overdoses, seizures, allergy, abdominal pain, asthma, collapsed lungs, or assault wounds (like the one I naughtily dubbed the 'Liverpool Lovebite', when a chunk of earlobe was bitten off).

Looking back, I was absurdly busy throughout that decade, working all the hours, compiling a hefty handbook for the department, publishing papers on our caseload, training staff and colleagues in and outside the hospital in resuscitation, trauma, toddler and toxicology care, running umpteen meetings, as well as the postgraduate medical education service for the Royal and its sister hospital, Broadgreen General. Still, the pleasure of working with so many great nurses, doctors, keen students of every kind, and all sorts of department staff sustained me. So too did being a newlywed and a father of one, then two, then three little girls, with 'names like a bad hand of Scrabble', as my Scottish brother-in-law described Ciara, Naoise and Aoibhe. And we gradually moved up the property ladder, from 'compact and bijou' in Orford Street, to relatively spacious suburban life in Middlefield Road, just off Menlove Avenue, which leads to the airport. This was two hundred yards down the road from the legendary Strawberry Fields, and four hundred yards up the road from No. 251 Menlove Avenue, where John Lennon had lived with his Aunt Mimi, and where his mother, Julia, was knocked down and killed. And in a way that was kind of magical for even a restrained fan, we lived exactly a mile from where Lennon first met McCartney.

I also slowly got into the swing of Liverpudlian theatricality. If Edinburgh had brought out the committed emergency physician in me, Liverpool was where I found myself becoming a sort of medical performance artist. I discovered that standing up in front of an audience, big or small, and talking about the stuff that interested, exercised or infuriated me, was something that really energised me. I began to imitate the enthusiasm and confidence of my former mentors in Edinburgh, Drs Little, Robertson and Steedman, who commanded the complete attention of their audiences as soon as they spoke, whether in the Back Theatre in the Royal Infirmary or on an international stage in London. In fact, they'd really kick-started the process by getting me to teach regularly at the Royal College in Edinburgh, the police headquarters, ambulance and mountain rescue team bases and at national conferences.

Lawrence called my approach 'infotainment' and I hope that I didn't become too messianic in the process, but I did remind myself that St Luke, the patron saint of artists and doctors, was often described in literature as a 'physician and evangelist'. That idea of the medic *evangelising* or trying to persuade others to believe in what the NHS was doing, what *we* were doing, became my explicit motivation. So I spoke to crowds of staff in the Royal's Grand Rounds, as well as to smaller audiences in the A&E department, GPs' and dentists' surgeries, the Liverpool Medical Institution, the Royal Army Medical Corps, trainees' groups and NHS management workshops. The more I spoke, the more I got invited to speak at other hospitals' Grand Rounds, or at national and international meetings around the UK, or to get involved in interesting new projects. And the more I enjoyed this performative part of medical life, the more I appreciated my brief time in DramSoc.

One initiative, of which I was quietly proud, was the Car Offender Programme (COP). This was a pioneering project run by the Merseyside Probation Service in partnership with, for instance, police driving instructors, bereaved families, the insurance industry and the A&E department at the Royal. In 1991, the Probation Service approached Lawrence and me to see if we would be interested in a pilot project aimed at recidivist (endlessly reoffending) car thieves, who kept coming up before the local magistrates again and again. They said they were trying to interrupt this vicious cycle, and I jumped at the idea, having encountered the scourge of joyriding while I was working in St James's in Dublin in 1983. Liverpool was suffering from an epidemic that was virtually identical to the one across the Irish Sea, and the recipe seemed to include the same ingredients: poverty, boredom due to an absence of things to occupy teens, alcohol and cannabis-driven apathy towards the consequences, parenting deficits and family breakdown. All these have been repeatedly itemised where joyriding exists.

I had absolutely no idea what to expect when I started my contribution to the COP in 1991, but I soon got the hang of it. Once a month, about a dozen young offenders were brought to our teaching room in the Royal, where I had set up my slide projector to project massively enlarged pictures of little finger wounds, minor cuts to faces, ankle sprains, and so on. The idea was to engage with the youngsters, to make them connect with the rollercoaster of stories I'd tell and to get their views on various scenarios or their suggestions as to what to do with a series of worsening injuries, culminating in the physically sickening. Invariably the young lads (I recall no girls) would come in throwing shapes but would leave throwing up. Or nearly doing so. But I was unapologetic about this approach, which I dubbed 'visual vaccination'. It was clear to me that these boys had had few or no father figures in their lives, or at least no adult male seemed ever to have taken their opinion seriously before. And almost every month, I saw these young men transformed from scary Scouse crims, the sort you'd cross the road to avoid, to the kind of clearly heartbroken boys who'd come from chaotic homes or had been 'in care', that most uncaring of starts. I saw for myself, time after time, what a little interest or encouragement, what people dismissively call 'attention', can do for these defiant but vulnerable lost souls. And even if I am a romantic ex-orphanage boy myself, the results of an independent study by the University of Liverpool of the impact of the week-long programme were encouraging. It seemed that the reoffending rate among the participating Merseyside offenders within a year of facing the magistrates was about 24 per cent, compared with a national Home Office average of 43 per cent. Better still, the effect wasn't dependent on one person, and my brilliant Irish colleague in Liverpool, Una Geary, achieved the same results when she took over the COP (and much else besides).

The COP confirmed for me how we, as medics, could perform other types of healthcare – preventive and pre-emptive. I was moving from a view of the A&E department as an endpoint, to the notion that you could, in fact, work back to the *causes* and try to stem the flow of patients that way. It was a compelling idea, and I began to seek out other ways to do this.

After a decade at the ever-busier medical frontline, I was forming stronger and stronger opinions on *why* people ended up in A&E and realising that we didn't just have to treat the result, we really *had* to try to intervene to treat the cause. Some might have argued that it was beyond our remit, but effective initiatives like the COP taught me otherwise. It also taught me that success breeds success. Other invitations to perform or contribute followed from the Home Office, Royal Colleges, various special interest groups, Waterloo RFC, the BBC, the *Big Issue* and the 'corporate' NHS. But some of the most enticing turned out to be from colleagues in the Drug Services in Liverpool, with whom I collaborated in creating a novel substance misuse module for medical undergraduates and in the production of a safer injecting guide, by Jon Derricott and others, which I'm delighted to say remains a key reference for Merchants Quay Ireland.

Easily the most alluring invite though, for a former party animal, was an approach by the management of Cream, the famous superclub that was located in a particularly derelict part of the city, Wolstenholme Square. In fact, it was one of the city's musical legends, Jayne Casey, who came up with the proposal. In the 1970s, Jayne, as charismatic and fabulous a Scouser as you're likely to find, had been the shaven-headed lead singer in the famous Liverpool punk band Big in Japan, with Holly Johnson, Bill Drummond, Ian Broudie and Budgie, all of whom went on to top the charts in bands like Frankie Goes to Hollywood and The Lightning Seeds. When I met her in 1992, Jayne was working with Cream on its marketing side and she came to meet me at the Royal to see if there might be an opportunity to collaborate with the club and the police in making it a safer venue. Cream had been extraordinarily successful in its first few years, but the usual trouble had started in the form of gangs, drug-dealing and threats at the door. The club's founders, James Barton, Darren Hughes and Andy Carroll, had made a truly unusual decision to reach out to the local constabulary and medics to see what might be done to avoid a future terminal encounter with the law or licensing authorities.

In practice, the medical part meant me visiting the club during the daytime to discuss its 'customer care', and then during a busy night as thousands of customers partied within its cavernous confines. I remember being led through the packed club by Claire Lambe, the manager, and finding it utterly different from the sticky-floored venues of my youth in Ireland. I was mesmerised by the connected series of huge rooms, each with a different genre of equally deafening music (Balearic, House, Acid, etc.) and astounding lighting and special effects. But what impressed me most was the lack of aggression and the absence of violence. I wasn't the only one, it seems, as many people used to comment on the 'peaceful vibe' at Cream, which added to its remarkable global popularity. In fact, people regularly travelled from Dublin, Cork, Reykjavik, Amsterdam and New York to enjoy the atmosphere, and the sets played by DJs like Paul Bleasdale, Paul Oakenfold, Pete Tong, Sasha and Judge Jules.

I have little doubt that part of the explanation was the widespread consumption of the 'empathogenic' ecstasy, or E, which dominated youth culture in the UK at the time. It was notorious for randomly and pitilessly killing young users, but on the other hand it lacked the association with violence of so many other intoxicants. Of course, there were other factors in Cream's reputation, including a notoriously tough door policy. Anyhow, avoiding preconceptions as far as possible, myself, Cream's affable first-aider, the late Dave 'F.A.' McGreevy, Howard Morris, the Royal A&E department's even more amiable auditor-in-chief, my colleague Colin Dewar, and others undertook one of the first studies of how nightclubs affect an acute health service, like that provided at the Royal. We did so by scrutinising the caseload of the busy first-aid room at Cream, and the media absolutely loved some of the stuff we identified in the records.

On foot of our work and findings, in October 1997 the first *Club Health* conference was organised by Mark Bellis, Head of Public Health at Liverpool John Moores University, and his research associate, Mary Kilfoyle. It took place in the main room of Cream and they invited the legendary Tony Wilson, owner of the Hacienda nightclub and Factory Records in Manchester, to open the event with his views for an audience that included policymakers, politicians, public health specialists, clubbers and serious activists. Wilson's views were predictably strident, anti-establishment and dismissive of much of the government's so-called 'Reaganite bollocks', which he said sought to stop young people doing what they liked to do. His analysis of the club scene in the early 1990s was that it was an English working-class movement driven by youngsters returning from holidays in Ibiza, where they'd first savoured the electronic music and often ecstasy. He made sense when he talked of having free water, liberally available, and experienced security staff who knew when trouble was brewing, but even though the first ecstasy death in the UK had occurred in the Hacienda (the victim had taken the pill before she entered the venue), he seemed to think that flyers with health warnings were sufficient to prevent further health harm in clubs like his. As apparent 'proof' of this argument, he said he had not seen a single ecstasy-related death in Manchester in four years.

I spoke immediately after Wilson to the 250 people in the room. I described three years' first-aid workload in the club in which they were sitting, and I explained how half the problems seen in the first-aid room involved intoxication with alcohol or drugs, about a quarter were soft tissue injuries, and the rest involved a mixture of collapse, funny turn, panic attack or asthma. I estimated that about a million people went clubbing each weekend in the UK and the 'complications' of clubbing accounted for about 0.5 per cent of all A&E attendances each year. Such attendances amounted to about 25 million by 2019 in the UK, and 1.2 million in Ireland, so the number of sick and injured clubbers remains substantial. I also made the point that, while there was an almost infinite variety of hazards in and around clubs – from dark stairwells to slippery toilet tiles, broken glass to lasers in the eye, CS gas cannisters being lobbed into a crowd, and fireworks – only three really mattered in terms of scale. These were *criminality, cocaine and conflagration*. Interestingly, these remain the greatest dangers in nightclubs all over the world, in 2021, while alcohol remains the commonest 'proximate' or immediate cause of mishaps and malicious violence.

Inevitably, though, it was the non-serious but colourful issues in my talk that grabbed the attention of the tabloids, glossy magazines and radio shows over the next year or so. These included 'Nightclub Nipple' – the dancer's version of jogger's nipple, caused by chafing and cured by Vaseline. 'PVC Bottom' was chafing of the nether regions in those who insist on dancing for hours in plastic costumes. 'Club Finger' was peculiar to males who bend down in the dark to flick away a cigarette butt from the sole of their runners, only to find a piece of glass has neatly incised their fingertip. 'Club Foot' was the female version of this, for those who danced barefoot. In fact, for quite a while we hogged the headlines and the airwaves, and I briefly became 'Dr Ecstasy' and 'the clubbing medic'. But whatever about the titillating coverage, we were all entirely serious about the public health aspects of the urban night-time economy.

Back then, and ever since, my view has been that clubbing is a source of great pleasure, which in turn is vital to our well-being. Therefore, the purpose of an alliance between public services, like police or healthcare providers, and club or super-pub owners is simple: to reduce the burden on the public sector with evidence-based measures in and around licensed premises, so the night-time economy flourishes and people can enjoy a really good night out and get home afterwards, safe and sound. In short, medical and nursing care are essential in every big club, concert venue or festival.

The *Club Health* conference went on to become a biennial worldwide event, and it has been bringing people who care about party animals together for over twenty years. Indeed, one of the great pleasures of my later professional career was helping to bring *Club Health* to Dublin Castle in 2017, to celebrate the 20th anniversary with many of the original gang, along with dynamic Irish newcomers like Dr Siobhan O'Brien Green of Trinity and Dr Sarah Morton of UCD. The future of the debate about night-time safety in Ireland, at least, is safe in their hands.

Meanwhile, the other kind of 'inner-city life' was also adding immensely to our workload at the Royal, especially that going on in our own backyard, as it were. Toxteth's turbulent history and the fact that it had long been among the top three boroughs in England with the most extreme socioeconomic deprivation meant that the area was a reliable source of work for the emergency department. For the most part, the cases from the Liverpool postcode L8 were genuinely accidental: trips, falls, or domestic misadventures that resulted in minor soft tissue trauma, head injuries or fractures. Some cases, however, could not be really classified as accidents, like the ghastly incident in October 1991 when a nine-year-old boy and twelve-year-old girl were killed by a joyrider as they crossed Granby Street, in Toxteth. But while assaults in the area continued to be ten-a-penny, fatalities from violence were relatively rare in the early 1990s, and deaths were usually the unintended consequence of a drunken or impetuous punch, kick or headbutt. Shootings did occur periodically, but they were often clumsy and intended targets were often missed.

And then came the great exception. The assassination of David Ungi, on 1 May 1995, was almost unique in its brutality, its slick execution and its ramifications. It was certainly the most memorable and significant murder during my decade in Liverpool. Ungi, a 36-year-old father of three, was a former boxing champion, who was described variously as a 'businessman' and an 'unemployed part-time used-car dealer'. He belonged to a family that was feared throughout South Liverpool and was used to being treated with respect, especially in their part of the city, which meant the Dingle side of Toxteth, on the river, and the city end of Aigburth Road, which was the location of a pub called Cheers, where everybody knew his name and what it signified. Or at least they did know, until the pub changed hands. And there the legends start to multiply.

The basic narrative is that a feud erupted between the Ungi family and another gang over the ownership of the pub and the Ungis' right to drink there. A 'straightener', or old-fashioned bare-knuckle fight, was arranged between Ungi and a man called John Phillips to settle the dispute. The contest took place on Byles Street and unsurprisingly, given his Golden Gloves pedigree, Ungi won, and he thought that was the end of the matter. But Phillips was far from finished, and he wasn't willing to accept defeat. Furiously alleging that Ungi had used a knuckleduster to clinch the contest, he reportedly ordered a hit on his rival. On the evening on 1 May, Ungi was driving along Toxteth's North Hill Street, in his VW Passat, when suddenly a black VW Golf GTi overtook him at speed, pulled in front of the Passat to block its progress, and a man jumped out brandishing an automatic weapon.

The gunman opened fire and 'at around 5.40pm, the father-of-three was hit twice, one of the bullets slicing straight through his main artery ... and he collapsed at the scene', according to later reports in the Liverpool Echo.

The shooting of David Ungi was later described as a watershed in the history of crime in Liverpool. It was also a momentous turning point in emergency medical care, one to which the truism applied: nothing would ever be the same again. Just two miles away, at the Royal, I was in my light-blue scrubs, halfway through my usual Monday evening shift. Although weary from the endless overcrowding in the department, I felt ready for almost anything that the night might throw at me. In those days, trauma, or serious injury, thoroughly excited me and I had personally invested a great deal in developing trauma management in the department. I was determined to drive the transformation of the Royal into a major trauma centre, with regular audits of our workload and advanced trauma life-support training for all the staff so they could respond in an effective and co-ordinated way to any kind of trauma. I'd also introduced what was a new type of monthly Trauma Forum, where all the many types of doctor, nurse and allied professional involved in caring for injured patients in the hospital (and in the whole Mersey region) could regularly scrutinise the Royal's management of injured patients, with guidance from experts of all sorts in trauma science. Of course, the most salient factor in trauma care, in my experience, is the quality of the staff, and I was certain in 1995 that we had some of the best nurses, doctors, radiographers and allied professionals in the world.

It can get very noisy as a patient is unloaded from an ambulance stretcher or spinal board onto the Resus trolley and orders are issued by the consultant or senior nurse to 'do this, find that, fetch the other, or track down the relevant specialist. Now!', while results of clinical measurement, blood tests or scans are called out, often repeatedly, in the hubbub. The ruckus is usually imperceptible to those busy doing what they're trained to do, following familiar drills or evidence-based protocols with zeal. Only the uninitiated or uninvited visitor perceives chaos, while a well-trained cardiac arrest or trauma team is usually 'in the zone' mentally, concentrating on the job at hand, oblivious to the outside world. But not on that May Day in 1995.

I have necessarily hazy memories of the events, but there were painful lessons that evening which I've never forgotten. The first was that gang warfare was both brutal and opportunistic, and the consequences for the emergency department were often unexpected as there was frequently little or no warning of the arrival of a shooting victim, as with Ungi. We only heard of his case when a brace of intensely anxious paramedics arrived into the department carrying the lifeless body, and breathlessly described the chaotic and frightening scenes around the victim's car, summarising what had happened. They recounted the simple but paralysing message roared in their faces by the victim's friends on North Hill Street: 'If he dies, you f—ing die!'

A basic mantra in emergency care is the self-explanatory *fail to prepare, prepare to fail*. If the victim of a shooting arrives without warning, there can be no preparation and you're on the back foot from the start. Given that emergency departments like the Royal are always busy and full of other patients needing critical care in the Resus Room, the response can be extremely fraught as a limited number of staff may have to deal with a cardiac arrest in one bay, a life-threatening meningitis in a second bay, and a gunshot victim in a third. In a nutshell, this sort of situation required enormous resilience and what might be described as an imperturbable zen-like mindset, on the part of senior clinical staff. Happily, by 1995 the staff at the Royal were used to dealing with all sorts of crisis in their well-designed facility, so there was minimal delay in getting to full throttle once the patient was delivered.

But − and this was the second lesson − what they were *not* used to was the subsequent banging on the Resus Room doors by the victim's distraught henchmen and extended family members, actually trying to break down the doors, despite the best efforts of security staff and the heavily armed police officers suddenly swarming around the department. The hospital photographer, who was involved regularly in recording clinical scenarios, for once declined my request − to take a photograph of the police sniper on the roof of a building across the street from the A&E department. His stress levels reflected those of most of the staff that night in Resus, where we felt genuinely as if we were in a siege situation.

Notwithstanding the anxiety, noise and minimal preparation, the response that evening was extraordinary, and came as close to a major incident response as anything else I saw in the 1990s. Within minutes, radical surgery was being undertaken in the Resus Room, and nurses, doctors, radiographers and specialists in anaesthesia, critical care, cardiology and thoracic surgery were summoned from all corners to contribute to the care of one critically injured individual. One thing was clear: we may not have been set up specifically to care for combat victims but, in my mind, we were as ready at that time as any civilian facility in the UK to manage severe gunshot trauma, and no life-saving intervention was withheld.

A third, unforgettable lesson that evening was that a bullet, a small ballistic missile, can cause devastating and hidden injury to the inside of a human body as it ricochets against bones and organs. And yet it may enter and exit the body through what look like trivial surface wounds. This means that, amidst the threats and intense anxiety of all staff, every conceivable intervention and every conceivable specialist may be required, within minutes, to deal with the reality as it is uncovered. Fortunately, every such specialist did work at the Royal.

The fourth and most dispiriting lesson of all is that, regardless of the superhuman efforts that may be put into saving the life of a shooting victim and regardless of the levels of resources and expertise available, many casualties cannot be revived due to the damage done to crucial parts of their anatomy, be it the brain, heart, big vessels, or spinal cord, the instant they are shot. In short, while the greatest emergency physician or surgeon can work miracles, the impossible remains just that.

I quickly learned all those painful lessons that night when, despite the heroic efforts of many of the hospital's first-class specialists, we realised that we could not save David Ungi's life. As they say in Liverpool when someone's luck runs out, 'There was nothing down for him'. But for those of us who had struggled in vain to revive him, there followed one final painful lesson, learned over time: fear and violence are extraordinarily contagious, and we should all be grateful for the bravery of the men and women in the police, and the security industry, who, like the medics and nurses in the A&E department that night, represent another very thin blue line.

The urban gang warfare in Liverpool in 1995 started symbolically, and none too subtly, a couple of days after the assassination with an arson attack on the pub, Cheers. Three days later a row of houses in Lydiate, in Halewood, was sprayed with gunfire. By Friday, 5 May, armed police in armoured vehicles were patrolling the streets of Liverpool, particularly in Toxteth. Eight days later a man was shot by two gunmen who burst into a gym in Beech Street. The police linked the shooting to the Ungi case. Thereafter the number of victims escalated rapidly: a 31-year-old man was shot in Netherley on 15 May, a 36-year-old man was shot in Dovecot, and on 20 May a man was shot five times in the city centre and a woman, an 'innocent passer-by', was shot in the hip. On 4 June, shots were fired into a house in Princes Avenue, in Toxteth, and on 8 June a man was shot in a doorway, also in Toxteth. Another man was shot in Moses Street, Toxteth, on 19 June and died five months later as a result. And on and on it went. More houses and cars were sprayed with bullets, other cars were torched, and teenagers affiliated with the opposing Ungi and Phillips sides were seen openly waving Uzi submachine guns around Toxteth.

At the Royal, the shooting cases just kept coming, and with each case police in flak jackets, cradling Heckler & Koch semi-automatic carbines, with Glock pistols in their holsters, arrived before, or sometimes with, the victim to patrol outside the emergency department's doors. Shocked at first, all of us began to take their visits for granted. One of the crew in reception reckoned there'd been ten separate shooting cases brought into us within three weeks of Ungi's death, but the truth was that we began to lose count.

What was clear was that each case was unique, they often arrived unexpectedly into the A&E department, and sheer luck played more of a role in the outcome than in any other condition I have ever encountered. One man, for instance, walked into the Triage room from the ambulance that had brought him to the hospital, complaining that he'd suddenly become deaf on his right side 'after a shooting in the pub' where he'd been drinking all day. The patient was plainly drunk but otherwise unperturbed, not just by the fact that a gun had been discharged behind him but by the ragged wound about his right ear, a tiny 'cut' just behind it, and the blood trickling from his right nostril. It was only the deafness that was annoying him, he told the nurse, and this had developed immediately after he'd heard 'a very loud bang'.

The nurse assessing him was not unduly concerned, given the unimpressive findings, but she arranged a skull x-ray, just in case. The x-ray looked normal, but half an hour after the patient arrived, the nurse received a message from the police at the scene who told her that a 9mm bullet had been found in the pub. It was suspected that the patient must have sustained a glancing blow from this, so he was admitted for observation and an Ear, Nose and Throat assessment the following morning. However, a few hours into his admission, the patient had a generalised convulsion, which necessitated a brain scan. It was this that revealed that the bullet had penetrated his skull just behind the right ear, and had emerged through his nostril, fracturing parts of the inner skull and the jaw joint during its passage.

A mixture of extraordinary luck and intoxication characterised that presentation, and we found that many of our shooting victims were similarly intoxicated with drink or drugs, or just evasive, making history-taking particularly difficult. Similarly, the trajectory of bullets was sometimes the result of a bad shot, not infrequently because the gunman was also befuddled by drink or drugs. At other times the bullet couldn't miss and, if it penetrated any part of someone's anatomy, it usually caused massive damage. The case of Paul Ogbuehi was an example. He was a 23-year-old who was shot just once in a house in Toxteth on 31 November 1995, following some kind of row. It was unclear whether the shooting was intended to kill him, but the single bullet had passed through his arm and into his abdomen, where the spinning missile fatally disrupted the internal organs. In the typically atypical fashion of gangland warfare, he was dumped shortly afterwards in the front seatwell of a small car parked outside a Toxteth terraced house, where a young single mother was bathing her baby. Less than ten minutes later, this woman was running into the emergency department, where I met her at the ambulance entrance, screaming, 'They've shot Paul! They've shot Paul! And he's in the car outside!'

What had happened was that the driver had banged on her front door and ordered her to take the victim to the 'ossie', as the hospital is known in Liverpool. Again, we did our very best for the unfortunate victim, but there was 'nothing down for him' either, that day. I must admit, all these years later, I have seldom seen a more authentic look of terror than on that poor young woman's face that afternoon, nor, as a father at the time of two very little girls, can I forget the fact that she had been alone in her house, bathing her tiny baby, when they banged on her front door.

I also confess that the gang warfare that kept throwing cases at us in the Royal, leading to a great deal of stress among staff members, was one of the factors that eventually persuaded me to return to Ireland. Indeed, in 1999, when I started work in Cork, I used to say that 'I've come from the future'. I was right to be pessimistic, because within a decade, all the street crime and the related massive consumption of drugs like cannabis, cocaine, ecstasy and even heroin, had reached every small town in Ireland. And with it, the Liverpool-style gang violence that I had hoped to escape.

As if to emphasise the comparison between the evolving situation in Ireland and the globalised and murderous drug trade in Liverpool, a suspected Brazilian hit squad was apprehended in the quiet rural village of Clara, in County Offaly, at the end of May 2020. Four men travelling in a van and a car were arrested and a search of the vehicles revealed a submachine gun, a shotgun and ammunition. It was reported that the Gardaí believed the South Americans were en route to Tullamore, to assassinate a member of 'a Traveller gang' involved in the drugs trade in the area. So my main worry now is that the necessary elements for a rapid spread of gangland killings, and all the inevitable collateral damage, are already in place in the UK, Ireland and many parts of the neighbouring continent. I see relatively few obstacles, given the enormous appetite for drugs and alcohol in these islands, and the enormous levels of intoxication, stress, dependence, mental health and greed generated by the sale and consumption of the main long-term and 'proximate' causes of violence – alcohol, amphetamines, benzodiazepines, cannabis and cocaine.

The greatest error, in my opinion, is to think that the cause is mainly people falling out over money. The cause of the violence lies within the cerebral limbic system of the people who consume these drugs and then become homicidally, irrationally, impulsively and recreationally violent. And, again in my humble opinion, the frontline staff in the country's emergency departments must not fail to prepare for the inevitable medical fallout, and for the contagion I first saw in Liverpool, of fear and ever-greater violence.

In July 2015, twenty years after the Ungi assassination, an 18-year-old teenager, riding on the back of a motorcycle on a South Liverpool Street, was shot dead with a 12-gauge shotgun, fired from the driver's window of an Audi A3. A few hours later, a policeman's body-camera recorded a video of Luke Kendrick, the 24-year-old owner of the car, bragging in his aunt's sitting room: 'Look what's happened now, mate, you're dead, ha ha ha ha ... I'm f—ing made up, stick that on the camera'.

The local press reported that the 'unstable and aggressive' Kendrick was subsequently found guilty of the teenager's murder, and he later grotesquely abused and mocked the deceased's family in court. His friend, Ryan Bate, was also found guilty of the killing. They were both sentenced to 24 years in prison. But it was never established who had fired the gun. A third man who had been in the Audi was not apprehended and fled abroad on the night of the murder. Described in newspapers as a 'baby-faced killer', he continues to appear on the UK's National Crime Agency Most Wanted posters in connection with the murder of Vinny Waddington, and 'the unlawful distribution of controlled drugs in the Liverpool area'.

His name? David Ungi, Junior.

The Leaving of Liverpool

By 1998, Liverpool was home to the Luke family, and we were all thriving there, in our lovely semi-detached 1930s house near Calderstones Park. But 'going home' for me still meant Ireland, and in August of that year, all the Lukes set out to pay a visit to our old family friends, Steve and Rosemary Cusack, and their children, in Cork. Steve and I had been medical school classmates in UCD and, in 1987, we'd found ourselves working as Registrars together at the Royal Infirmary in Edinburgh. There followed a couple of years of happy comradeship and socialising, but we'd then gone our separate ways, as medics do: me to Liverpool, and Steve to Glasgow to pursue further training, and then to Cork where he was a consultant at CUH. Invariably, the two families had much to discuss when we met up every few months, but this reunion turned out to be particularly memorable.

Driving from Dublin to Cork by the scenic route, along the Waterford coast road, we were all packed into the little Renault Clio that my mother had kindly lent us, and it really struggled to carry the weight of the five of us up the hill on the N20, just west of Dungarvan. We'd just crested the top, and the car had finally picked up some momentum going down the other side, when we were pulled over by a Garda and issued with a speeding fine (an 'on-the-spot fine to be paid within three weeks', as my Scottish wife sarcastically commented). So the mood in the car was somewhat subdued as we exited the village of Castlemartyr, in East Cork, keeping within the speed limit, at around 8.20 p.m. on a gorgeous late summer's evening.

Suddenly, on the Cork city side of the village, on the opposite side of the road, we saw a badly smashed and smoking Toyota Corolla, and a fire engine that had pulled up near it, whose crew were already out and assessing the scene. And some way off to our left was a black, high-powered Honda Integra, which had apparently ploughed into the back of the Toyota, at speed, and then ricocheted off into the long grass. I pulled over quickly, ran across the road to see what I could do, and found four occupants trapped behind the crumpled doors.

The crash had clearly happened only a matter of minutes previously and it was obvious that, while all the passengers were very seriously hurt, a boy of about eleven years of age was critically injured and semi-conscious. As I was assessing the situation, the fire brigade started to cut the passengers out, and shortly afterwards the first ambulance arrived at the scene. Given the scale of the situation, I shouted over to Vicky to help, and she took over the initial care of the most severely injured boy in the back of the first ambulance once he had been extricated. Bizarrely, one of the A&E trainees from the Royal in Liverpool, Brendan McCann (now a consultant in Waterford), also happened upon the scene. Dispensing with any small talk about the coincidence that had landed us both there, we found ourselves in the back of the ambulance doing what we could to halt the deterioration of the poor boy as the vehicle hurtled towards Cork. I had rung Steve within minutes of arriving at the scene and given him a brief summary of what had happened. I had asked him to 'activate the trauma team', or at least the surgeons, anaesthetists and radiologists and anyone else he cared to include, to be ready for our arrival at Cork University Hospital within 30 minutes or so.

Sadly, the young patient did not survive the devastating injuries he had sustained when the Honda ploughed into his mother's Toyota. He died a couple of hours later, despite the best efforts of the staff of CUH, who were indeed waiting in the emergency department as we brought him in. The poor family experienced a complete nightmare that evening as several of them were badly injured and were themselves transported to CUH in a second ambulance, to be treated by the assembled teams in Resus.

It transpired later that the Honda had been stolen in Youghal 40 minutes before the collision with the Toyota. Its 19-year-old driver immediately fled the scene and hid in the nearby Castlemartyr Woods, but he was caught by the Gardaí about four hours later. He turned out to be a serial joyrider, with a chaotic back story, who had already spent eight years in a children's detention centre for car theft and other crimes. While the young man was subsequently jailed for ten years for causing the lethal crash, he served just five years of that sentence. In 2013 he triggered another high-speed Garda chase while on a drunken spree in a stolen BMW.

It's hardly surprising that the girls never forgot what happened that night, as they were locked into our little car while my wife and I both did what we could on the side of the road. I often wondered if that was when Ciara Luke got the 'bug' for the career in emergency and critical care medicine she subsequently pursued. And I'd like to think she was equally impressed with her mother, who had raced into action, even though she had been away from emergency nursing at that stage for a few years. Anyway, after the ambulances had left the crash site outside Castlemartyr, Vicky drove on to our hosts' house, and Steve and I joined her and Rosemary an hour or so later. And later still, *chez* Cusack, after the three Luke girls had been lifted into bed, Steve marvelled over a late dinner at how I'd 'put the whole of CUH on alert' for the case. And he wondered if I could make a 'slightly less dramatic entrance next time, please'.

It was that night that I saw for myself that pre-hospital and trauma care in Ireland had a way to go yet, but my ambition to get home was nonetheless intensified. I knew that I was determined to be part of the process of bringing about a transformation in emergency medical care in my home country, and to bring back the knowledge and skills I'd acquired in Liverpool, Edinburgh and Australia. But translating all this into an actual move back to Ireland would involve much more than wishful thinking. After all, the reason I'd had to leave Ireland in the 1980s was the shortage of posts in the health service, at every level. And it wasn't that I wasn't keen. I'd been writing to former consultant bosses in Irish hospitals almost since the day I'd left in 1986, but less than a handful of jobs in emergency medicine were advertised in the following decade. So, I waited.

I was told again and again to 'press on' by a sympathetic Frank Ward in St James's, and to 'be patient, Chris!' by the ever-upbeat John Fennell in Dublin, and others, as they kept an eye out for me for a suitable post. And I had been patient, exceptionally so. I'd taken up a consultant post in Liverpool, worked diligently to develop the Royal's emergency and education services, seen three daughters born, and moved house twice, all the while waiting and hoping for an opportunity to move home. But now, as I approached 40, I was becoming anxious that the window was closing. In truth, while I was well established in the Royal and had received 'merit points' (with a small financial bonus) for my contribution to the NHS, I was grappling mentally with the early features of burnout, and physically with a hectic emergency department workload.

Even though there had been a significant growth in the size of the specialty in the UK, which by then had the third-highest number of consultants across all NHS disciplines, the problem was that the more we did, the more we were expected to do. The workload and the level of responsibility weighed heavily on all of us. It demanded a level of mental and physical stamina that simply couldn't be sustained – especially as the A&E department got busier and busier over those years. During my early years at the Royal, I used to stand in the nurses' station every now and then and shout, 'Are there any don't-care assistants around?!' And my motto in the first few years of consultancy had been, 'Without stress, my life has no meaning!' Oh, how we used to laugh.

But the abiding clinical memory of my final year at the Royal was of standing despondently one teatime in the mayhem in the A&E department, in between cardiac arrest and trauma calls to Resus, and deciding I had to call in the consultant physician 'on-take' for that evening and ask for his help in processing the huge numbers of patients awaiting

admission to wards, under *his* care. I popped upstairs to my
office, just above Resus, and rang him at home. I still recall
how shocked he seemed to be when I explained why I was
calling him. His terse response was, 'Okay, Chris, I'll come in,
but just this once, mind you.' And he did, not long afterwards,
although not to see or sort any patients. He had come to see
and sort *me* out, it seemed. He asked if we could have a quiet
chat, and politely but firmly made it clear that he had no
intention of coming into the hospital 'out-of-hours' to clear
queues of patients, or anything of the sort. I was genuinely
flabbergasted, given that so many of the patients on trolleys
were 'his', and I was trying to digest what he was saying when
a call went out for the third cardiac arrest of the day. I had to
hurry away to Resus, and that was the end of the conversation.
But I still recall him saying, 'Keep up the good work, Chris!'
as I headed back into the fray.

My own once-a-week late evening shopfloor shifts were
'discretionary', not obligatory, but I really believed that it was
vital for the department staff to see us consultants as more
than just nine-to-fivers. All five consultants in the department
were working flat out, but we were simply not adequately
staffed for the volume of cases we were seeing every day of
the year. Nor were we really getting the recognition from the
management or other colleagues for the quantity or quality of
work we were doing.

Throughout the 1990s, we had gradually taken over the
care of many sorts of cases that fell between stools in the
hospital, like poisonings, head injuries, collapsed lungs, allergy,
asthma flares, seizures, complications of alcohol misuse, chest
pain, abdominal pain, and the care of the homeless. The fact
was that we were managing – or minding – hundreds of

such cases every year in our observation ward, and we were becoming quite expert at it, harnessing experience and the scientific evidence base for treatment.

In some ways, I was gratified by this, as we steadily reduced the length of hospital stay for conditions like pneumothorax (collapsed lung), mainly by sticking to the guidelines set out in our teaching programme and handbook. I was even more delighted when we managed to appoint dedicated specialist staff, like Lynn Owens, an alcohol specialist nurse, who went on to transform alcohol care throughout the UK, or Howard Morris, who put his BBC training to good use as the auditor of injury cases in the department, and whose analysis helped to propel the Royal into the top ranks of trauma hospitals in the UK. Their friendship was just as important, of course, as their work, and it was our collective sense of playing for the team which kept us all going.

But, from my point of view, 1999 was a tough year, when I needed all the friends I could get. In one sense I was a victim of my own success in terms of the nightclub medicine, car offender, alcohol, drug, trauma and education projects. I was invited to give talks around the UK, to offer my views on drug issues to the Home Office, to lecture at the medical Royal Colleges in London, to join working parties and the Editorial Board of the *Journal of A&E Medicine*, to be the 'poster boy' of a safe city campaign in Liverpool (Operation Crystal Clear), and to contribute to various journals, from the *Nursing Times* to *CPD Anaesthesia* via the *Big Issue*. And there were certainly interesting aspects of such invitations, like working with the police and the big medicolegal law firms on drug-related deaths in custody, which fuelled my subsequent interest in cocaine (arguably as treacherous a drug

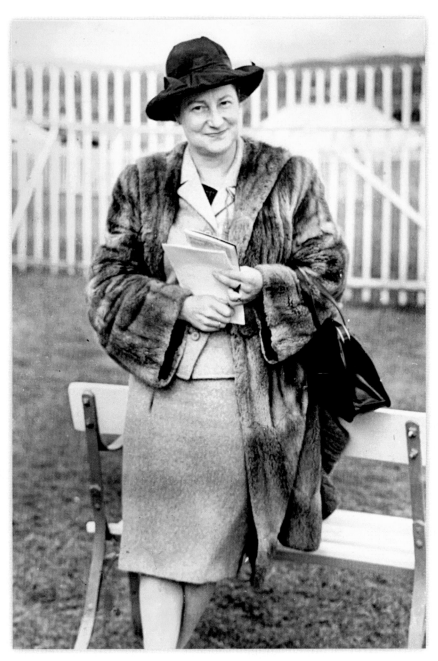

My mother, Colette Redmond: young, free and single, at the Curragh
Races in the 1950s.

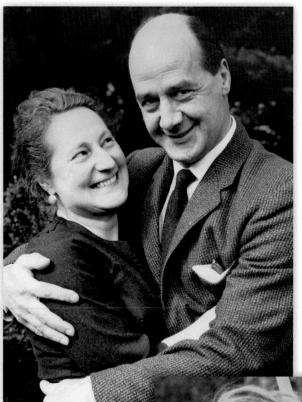

My mother and
father, Leslie Luke,
photographed c. 1962,
in the garden of
No. 33 Oaktree Road,
Stillorgan, Co. Dublin.

Me, aged c. 3 years old
on a visit to No. 33
from St Philomena's.

Me, aged c. 10 years old in my school uniform.

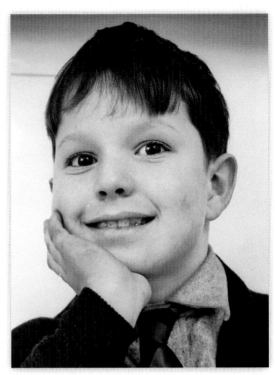

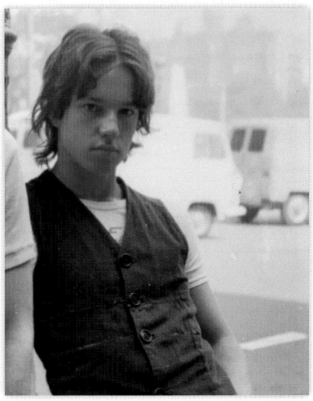

Me, aged c. 16 years, after hitching to Barcelona.

Graduating from UCD's School of Medicine in June 1982.

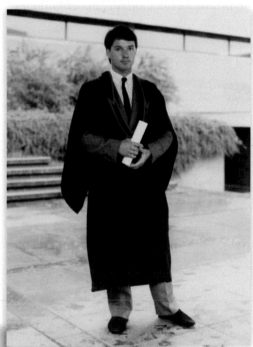

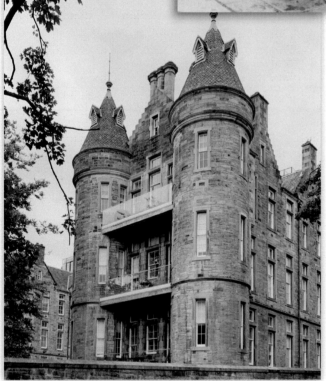

The Royal Infirmary of Edinburgh, which was designed in line with Florence Nightingale's 'pavilion' layout.

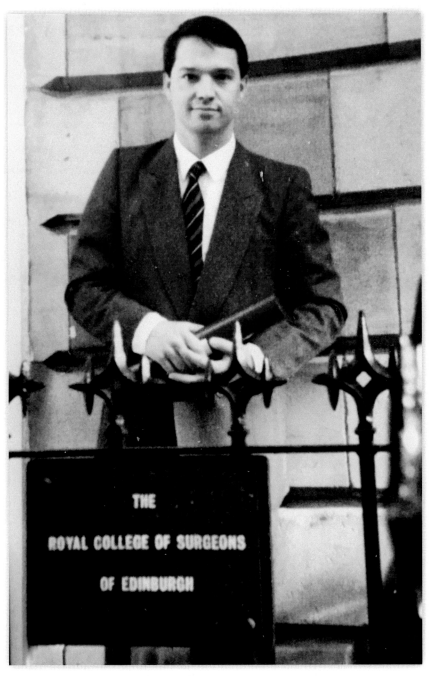

Me, aged c. 28 years, on Fellowship Day at the Royal College of Surgeons of Edinburgh, 1987.

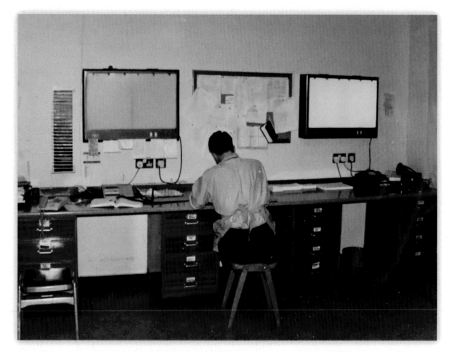

Working as a registrar in the Ambulatory 'Exam' Section, within the Royal Infirmary of Edinburgh's A&E department, c. 1989.

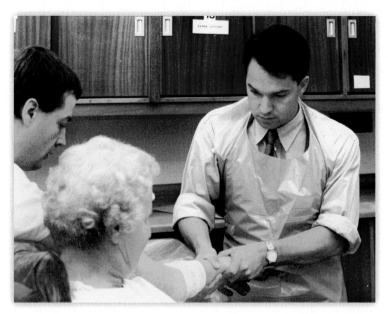

Manipulating a wrist fracture under regional anaesthesia, within the A&E department of the Royal Infirmary of Edinburgh, c. 1989.

My final shift as a registrar in Edinburgh, during which I was treated to a traditional farewell 'flour shower', c. 1989 (with nurses Paula, Pauline, Lorna, and Shona).

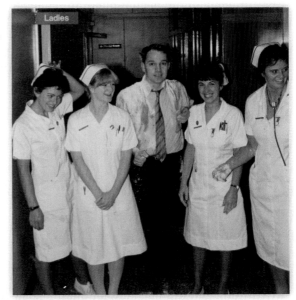

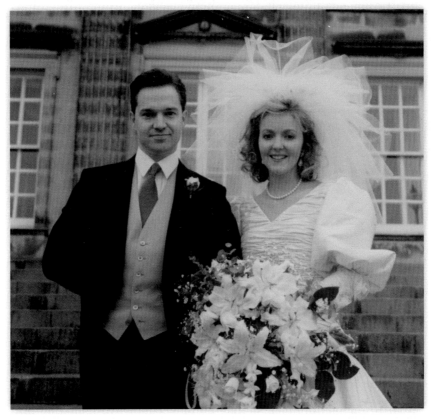

The new Mr and Mrs Luke: with Victoria on our wedding day, on the steps of Hopetoun House near Edinburgh, 1990.

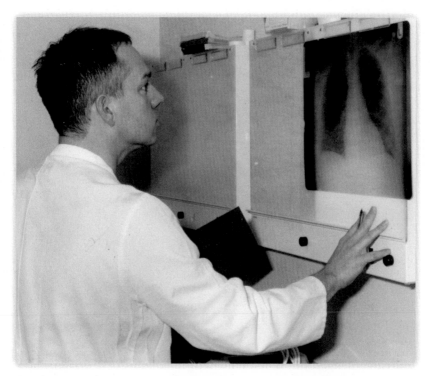

Inspecting a chest x-ray at the Royal in Liverpool, 1992.

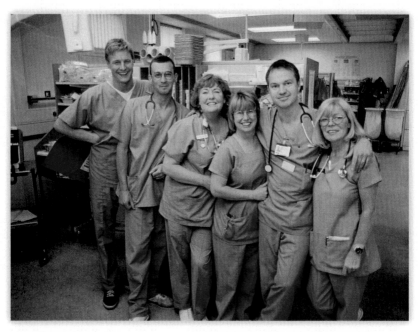

With the Royal Resus Team in 1998: Jamie, Allan, Josie, Anne and Cathy.

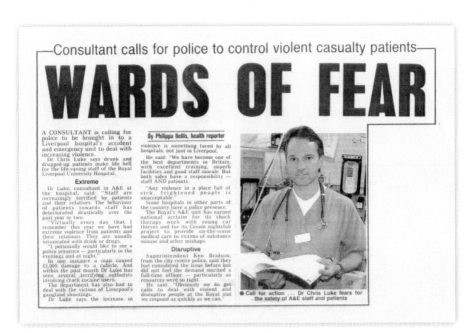

Newspaper headline as violence increased in Liverpool's A&E: 'Wards of Fear', 1994. (*Courtesy of the* Liverpool Echo)

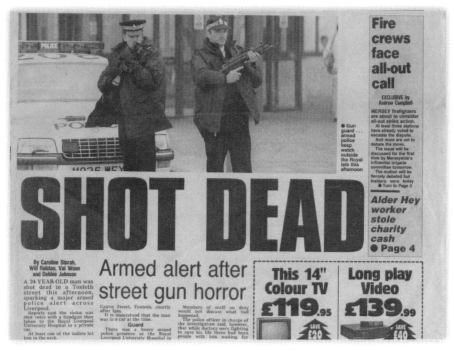

Newspaper headline referencing Liverpool's escalating gang warfare: 'Shot Dead', 1995. (*Courtesy of the* Liverpool Echo)

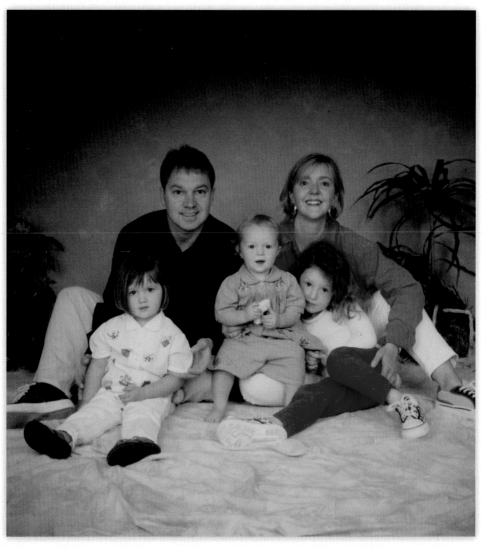
The Luke family, c. 1999 (L–R: Naoise, me, Aoibhe, Victoria and Ciara).

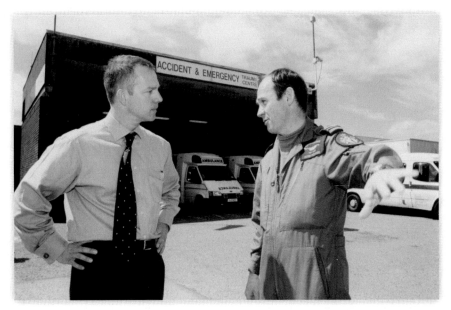

Meeting with a Royal Naval Air Squadron pilot, outside the old Cork University Hospital ED, c. 2000.

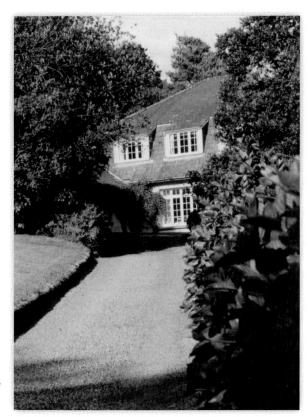

'Park House', our refuge in Castle Mary, east Cork. c. 2001.

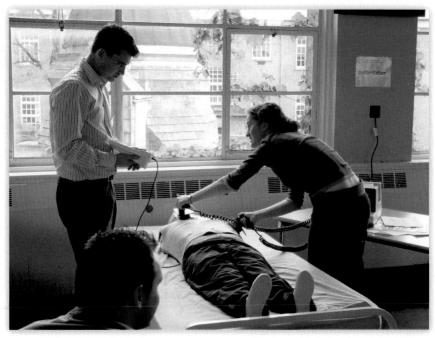

A young Dr Conor Deasy instructing on the pioneering UCC Final MB Clinical Skills course, 2005.

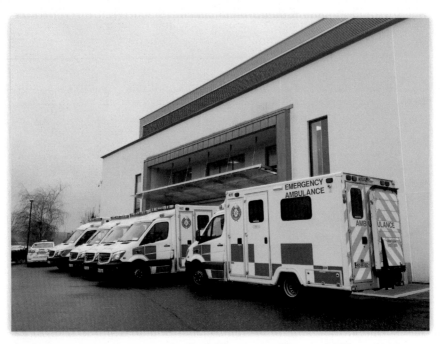

Ambulances queueing outside Cork University Hospital ED, c. 2018.

Burnout is greatest threat to health service, top medic warns

Evelyn Ring

Burnout is the greatest threat of all to the health service, according to one of the country's leading emergency physicians, Dr Chris Luke, who has announced he is stepping down from his current position.

Dr Luke, who works at Cork University Hospital and Mercy University Hospital, said he is withdrawing from the frontline after 35 years due to a health issue.

A form of arthritis in his neck has caused some nerve damage that affects his right hand so he has decided to retire early from his position.

He said he hopes to remain in healthcare and, as a fanatical radio listener, has an interest in broadcasting.

In an interview with Miriam O'Callaghan on RTÉ radio, Dr Luke said the greatest challenge in the health service in the English-speaking world is burnout.

He said burnout is a form of "spiritual anaemia" — the exhaustion of the spirit — and it is that kind of energy that sustains the health service. The British and Irish health services are predicated on the heroic doctor model but sometimes it is not enough for a doctor or a nurse to be heroic.

"Can I say to the powers that be that burnout is truly the greatest threat of all because the loss of that energy and that vocation is far more nefarious than the want of beds or staff," he said.

Dr Luke said that while the health service in Ireland has improved because of advances in science and technology, there are not enough beds and there are problems recruiting staff because the conditions are challenging.

He recalled sitting outside a post office in Stillorgan, Dublin, during the summer heatwave in 1976 and having two letters in his hands.

One was a letter to the Law Faculty in Trinity College Dublin and the other was to the School of Medicine in University College Dublin.

"I suppose I came up with the idea that medicine was a noble, self-sacrificing enterprise and, on balance, it gave me a bit more security — that's what nudged it."

Dr Luke said the sudden death of his father when he was a small child affected him hugely.

His mother worked at St James's Gate Brewery. He was an only child and spent a lot of time on his own.

However, he had a happy 12 years in St Conleth's College in Ballsbridge where he became a school captain.

Dr Luke said his maternal grandmother had grown up in the tenements in Gardiner St in Dublin. "It was only when we studied the census that we found that she started life in the tenements. And I know she had a really difficult time. Her father was an army man and he had mental issues."

Dr Luke said he often told colleagues working in inner-city hospital emergency departments that "difficulty makes people difficult".

"If you are wondering why this person drinks too much or smokes too much or has a generally chaotic life, remember that their privation and emotional difficulties will make them difficult in turn to deal with."

Asked why he chose emergency medicine, Dr Luke said it was his time in Moze in Zambia in the early 1980s that helped him make up his mind.

He worked in a bush hospital with Sr Lucy O'Brien just after President Robert Mugabe won the war of independence. Sr O'Brien was a member of the Missionary Sisters of the Holy Rosary as well as a highly qualified physician and gynaecologist.

"We got to do all sorts of extraordinary things in terms of surgery and medicine," he recalled.

Dr Luke, a father of four, met his wife, Victoria, in the back of an ambulance when working in the Royal Infirmary in Edinburgh. He later moved to the Royal Liverpool University Hospital.

However, he was drawn back to Ireland by the need to mind his mother, who will celebrate her 95th birthday next month.

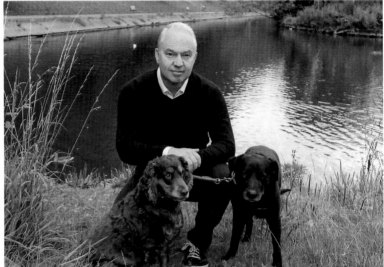

Dr Chris Luke, with his dogs Ruby and Ramsey. Speaking on RTÉ radio, he said: 'Can I say to the powers that be that burnout is truly the greatest threat of all because the loss of that energy and that vocation is far more nefarious than the want of beds or staff.' Picture: David Keane

With our family dogs, Ruby and Ramsay; newspaper headline about the burnout threat in healthcare, 2018. (*Courtesy of the* Irish Examiner)

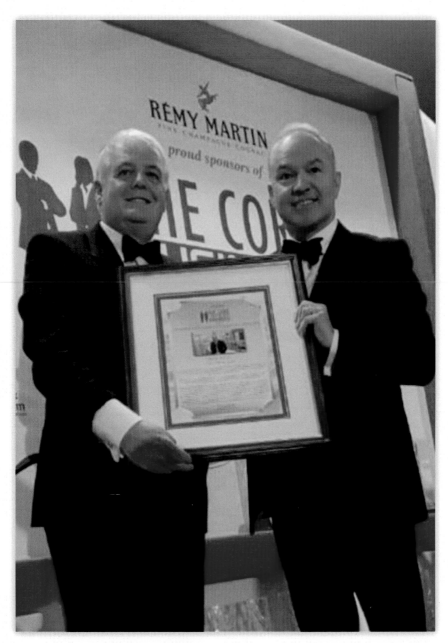

Receiving an award from John Minihan for my 'exceptional contributions to emergency medicine in Cork', 2018.

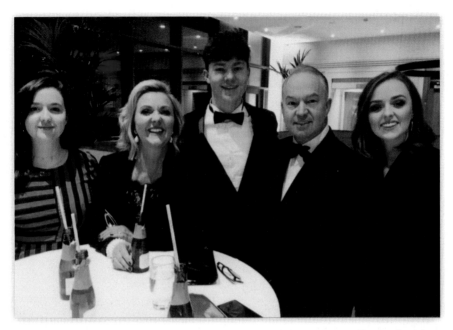

Five-sixths of the Luke family at the 2018 award ceremony (L–R: Aoibhe, Victoria, Harrison, me and Naoise).

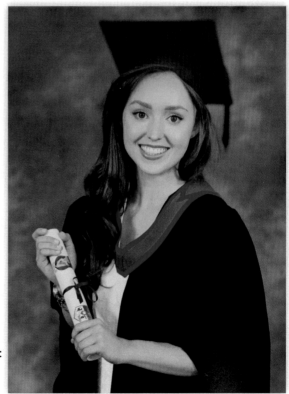

The next generation: Dr Ciara Luke on her graduation day.

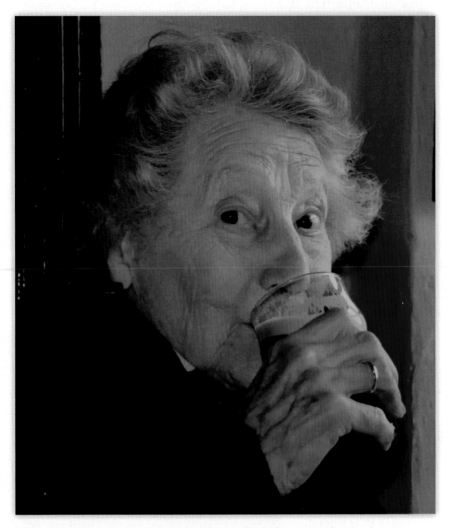

In her nineties, my mother sips a drop of her favourite drink: the 'black stuff'.

as alcohol when it comes to sudden medical and forensic calamities).

The latter was to become a particular interest of mine as I became involved in cases of sudden cocaine-related deaths in custody. Even as a medic with considerable experience of street drugs by then, I was taken aback as I discovered the way that the 'Bolivian marching powder' could so often kill even the most seasoned users.

In practice, the most notorious deaths occurred in people who had been arrested in a drugs bust or for behaving erratically or aggressively on the street. The classic story was that the police officers would be pretty sure that the user had stuffed a wrap of the drug into their mouths as soon as they anticipated arrest, but the user (and often his companions) would completely deny possession of any drug. So it was only ten or fifteen minutes later, in the police station, that the 'stuffer' went from aggressively protesting his innocence to gradually becoming unconscious in the cell, and then starting to convulse violently. The basic cause was the slightly delayed absorption of the cocaine as it reached the stomach and beyond, and the levels of the drug in the bloodstream surged to levels associated with intense aggression, then generalised seizure, stroke or cardiac arrest. And, of course, experts will realise that a cardiac arrest and a convulsion can look much the same to begin with, just to add to the diabolical complexity of the problem. This is a pretty familiar scene in police stations in cities where cocaine is used recreationally, and it's hard to know how to deal with the issue because, unless the victim is massively and urgently sedated, cocaine poisoning can trigger a fatal downward spiral for which there are shockingly few remedies. You could of course suggest education or legislation (the usual 'answers'), but the biology of cocaine means that users are often extremely sure of themselves, their rights and opinions until they're lying, convulsing, in the corner of a dining room, dancefloor or police cell.

On the personal side, in 1999 my oldest daughter was approaching her eighth birthday, and I had sort of decided that once she reached ten years of age, I wouldn't be able to justify moving her from her place of birth, her primary school and her local children's hospital, Alder Hey, where she was doing okay – or at least not doing too badly, despite being on chemotherapy and massive doses of steroids for a severe kidney condition. My primary concern, though, was my mother, who was then approaching 80 and living on her own in Stillorgan, even if she was back and forth to Liverpool for visits and vice versa. She was remarkably robust, socially active and self-reliant, but I knew that this must be a time-limited situation, and I was all too aware that she was often lonely. I was her only offspring, and I was very anxious to be nearer to her in her eventual 'dotage'.

Then, finally, I saw the job advertisement that looked like my path home.

In early 1999, a consultant post was offered in Cork, covering (or working part-time in) three separate emergency departments – in the Mercy Hospital, in Cork University Hospital (CUH) and in the South Infirmary. It looked like a seriously challenging job in terms of workload and logistics, but I knew this was a rare, unique and unmissable opportunity to get back to Ireland. At that time, literally no one knew exactly when another post might come up, so for me there was a very real sense of 'now or never'. And so I decided to make one last concerted effort to get home, although not at any cost. After all, my Scottish wife missed her folks in Edinburgh, our other home from home, and moving to Ireland effectively meant emigration for her. We discussed the issue over and over, and Vicky nobly and generously agreed that I should go for it.

Once the decision was made, I focused on pursuing the post in Cork. This meant sending off, in February 1999, a complicated, highly detailed application form to the Local Appointments Commission, including all my previous medical posts, my vaccination status, qualifications, publications and referees, my Inter Cert and Leaving Cert results, and a comprehensive twenty-page CV. I also visited Cork in March to meet with Steve and a couple of consultants – Vinnie McDermott at the Bon Secours Hospital in Cork, who I'd known from Edinburgh, and Mark Phelan at the South Infirmary, who I'd first met at the Royal in 1989. I made it my business to meet with a wide range of people within healthcare in Cork, including Tony McNamara, the General Manager at CUH, the General Managers and senior consultants of the Mercy and South Infirmary, the Chief Ambulance Officer, Peter Curley, and the two nursing leads in the emergency departments at CUH and the South Infirmary, Sheila Wall and Phil McKenna. In total, I think I met with about eighteen people in Cork over two days. I studied the medical press on both sides of the Irish Sea, to analyse the general trends in healthcare, and in emergency departments in particular. I rooted out seventeen years' worth of Medical Council registration certificates, original diplomas and reference letters from every hospital in Ireland where I'd worked, I wrote to five potential professional referees, and I obtained a letter of good standing from my medical indemnity or insurance provider, the Medical Protection

Society (confirming that I'd not been struck off or censured in any lawsuits).

I also studied the relevant official literature: the Report of the Commission on Nursing, the Report of the Review Group on Accident and Emergency Medicine Services in Cork for the Southern Health Board, the latest strategy of *Comhairle na nOspidéal* (the statutory body that regulated consultant appointments), the resourcing of the three emergency departments in Cork, and I composed a SWOT analysis. I even returned to Cork on a flying one-day visit at the end of April, to meet with Nuala Coughlan and Anne Hennessy, the lead A&E nurses at the South Infirmary and Mercy, as well as other senior staff I hadn't managed to see in March. Last, but not least, I studied the 'opposition' – the eight other candidates for the post – as carefully as any football manager or chess player might do. I concluded that at least three of them would be major rivals for the post.

And so, on 12 May 1999, after a medical on Morehampton Road to assess my health and fitness, I turned up for interview at the Local Appointment Commission, near the Grand Canal in Dublin. Steve Cusack later told me that he couldn't believe how 'shattered' I looked as I sat before the panel of umpteen interviewers. Pale, exhausted and stammering, he said I looked like I was going to collapse any minute. But that was my usual health status by then and, thankfully, as with many a pale and wan patient, a glass of cold water worked wonders. I slowly got into my stride, resorting to every rhetorical device in the book, as Professor Plunkett from St James's, one of the panellists, attested afterwards. Steve recounted much later that the chairwoman said just one word as I left the interview room: 'Wow!' He said that my intense preparation had paid off, as had my patience, but now I still had to wait to find out if I'd done enough.

While I waited, the Royal A&E department was as busy as ever. I didn't regret my decision because even though I enjoyed – and was nurtured by – the affection of so many people in the Royal and the wider city, I knew that I'd also been seriously corroded by my decade on Merseyside, and I needed to move on. Most of this was due to the perpetual busyness of the Liverpool department, even if it was always offset by the brilliant and effervescent staff.

But no amount of joshing or banter could compensate for some highly personal events, like my young wife's miscarriage over Christmas 1990, when I found myself not just on duty in a hectic A&E department but also wheeling my own poor spouse into the operating theatre on the ground floor of the hospital. Then there had been the hideous events of 1993, in which two ten-year-old boys had abducted the two-year-old Jamie Bulger from a Bootle shopping centre and tortured him to death on a nearby railway line. That ghastly affair had garnered worldwide attention of the worst sort, and it cast a terrible pall over the city, just as it was recovering from the Hillsborough stadium disaster in 1989 (which had initially been blamed on the very Liverpool supporters who'd died in such numbers). I remember sharing the sense of shame of the entire citizenry following the monstrous Bulger crime. It fed into a perception that the city was seen by the outside world as an almost irredeemable lost cause. A bit like Northern Ireland in the decades before. And I have no doubt that there must have been a terrible burden of mental ill-health in the city during those years.

The growing gloom inside the Royal had been eased somewhat by the boost provided when the new A&E

department was built in 1994, but the ever-growing workload, threats to the staff and gang warfare had inevitably made life inside extraordinarily difficult. And, by the latter part of the 1990s, like many of the staff, I felt abandoned by the system, and I regularly contributed to the local and national media on the whole subject of emergency department overcrowding, its causes and effects. And, of course, regardless of my activities across the Irish Sea, I found myself getting ever busier at the Royal as 1999 went on, battling the chaos in the A&E department as well as touring lecture theatres, lawyers' offices and municipal buildings to honour educational, medicolegal and public health commitments.

And then, suddenly, weeks after my interview in Dublin, the leaving of Liverpool turned from a notion to a real prospect. On 2 July 1999, a letter arrived for me at the Royal, from the Chief Executive Officer of the Southern Health Board, informing me that I had been 'recommended by the Local Appointments Commission for appointment to the office of' Consultant in Accident and Emergency Medicine at CUH, the Mercy Hospital and the South Infirmary in Cork, and conveying his congratulations on my success.

I wasn't long in accepting the invitation and tendering my resignation to the Chief Executive of the Royal. And in July 1999, I made the front page of the *Liverpool Evening Echo* for the last time, under the headline: 'Top Doc Quits Over Huge Workload', which was one interpretation.

The relief of knowing I would finally be back living on the same island as my elderly mother was tinged with immense sadness at the prospect of leaving so many close friends behind. It wasn't just the crew at the Royal, but also the extracurricular Scouse mates too, like Brian O'Connor and his wife, Celia. Brian was the GP who had first paid a home visit to my wife, the 'mad blonde Scotswoman of Orford Street', as he described her, during her pregnancy with Ciara, and he and Celia, a microbiologist at the Royal, had become our first best friends in Liverpool, as the two families went on to have three offspring each during the 1990s. And then there were Jon and Chrissie Nelson, our neighbours in Middlefield Road, our next best friends. Along with their own two boys, they practically reared Ciara Luke, who always preferred to recuperate in their home when she got out of Alder Hey. And there were many other friends and neighbours in the city who we would miss terribly.

My colleagues at the Royal were a different matter. They were 'family' and I hated the idea that I was deserting them. In truth, I dithered over the announcement until, in the end, Pauline McGorrin, the effervescent A&E secretary, nudged me over the line with a note that captured the Scouse humour and affection that had kept me going at the Royal, year after year:

> *Dear CL, I know you are worried about telling your nursies [sic] and they may feel abandoned, etc, but I really feel you are misjudging them. There will be tears and so on ... that is to be expected, but only because everyone will be sorry to see you go.... you have given enough for this department – they know that and they will wish you well ... Anyway, I think you will miss us more than we miss you. Cork will be full of chaotic Irishmen, you will not be noticed there, and the secretaries will have been brought up on Irish charm and will be quite inured to it!*

The Irish talk of a stiff upper lip among the English, but of course when you get to know them, it is a different matter. And after ten years serving the people of Liverpool (arguably a separate nation, I know), I was in a position to judge. In short, 'when they were good, they were very, very good, and when they were bad, they were horrid'. A bit like the Irish, and the Scots. And when they became your friend, it was as much a cause for celebration as across the Irish Sea.

Lawrence Jaffey, my consultant colleague, was one such case. He and I had been wary of each other when I'd arrived in 1989, and there was lots of boyish rivalry and joshing. Lawrence had subsequently appointed me as a colleague in 1992, and he was one of those really great mentors, and friends, who has been like a big brother to me. He was good enough to give me a copy of his reference for me for the Cork job, which I kept, primarily for sentimental reasons, but also to document that fleeting moment when, as a medic, I may just possibly have been in my prime. For an Englishman, he was remarkably unreserved in his praise for my 'clinical skills, energy, vision' and he called me a 'great teacher', who had 'completely revolutionized postgraduate medical education' at the hospital. But what I cherished most, oddly, was the sentimental judgement: 'Chris is a charming and immensely likeable man who has an ability to get on well with colleagues at all levels and is invariably loved by his patients. In my capacity as Clinical Director, I receive more letters of appreciation that are directed at him than any other member of staff, and I have never received any complaints about his attitude or approach from anybody'.

In later years, when I experienced the very worst of gaslighting and a total collapse in self-confidence, those words were to sustain me. And, in turn, I've made a point of giving trainees and colleagues a copy of particularly enthusiastic references. I still think these can be the most important, meaningful and reassuring metrics in a medic's career.

I was giving up a lot by leaving Liverpool, as were all the rest of the Lukes, but, by way of compensation, there was a wonderful departure-fest for me and Victoria, with farewell dinner parties, a big departmental leaving-do in the trendy Life bar on Bold Street, a soiree for friends in the venerable Artists' Club and a special party on the mezzanine floor of Cream, on our last Saturday night in the city, 13 November 1999.

And that was it. A decade in the 'Pool of Life' was over and, on the week of 15 November 1999, the Luke family moved to Cork.

Three for the Price of One

O ne of my favourite Scouse colleagues in the Royal was Christine Kennedy, the glamorous and dynamic nurse manager in the A&E department. One of her pet sayings was, 'Which part of "no" do you *not* understand?' This was intoned with theatrically pursed lips, crossed eyes and an exaggerated Liverpudlian drawl. It was guaranteed to crack me up. Unfortunately, in reality, it is sometimes difficult, and occasionally impossible, to say *No* at work. I would have loved to have said it regularly in my first year back in Ireland, but there were compelling reasons why I could not.

First, there was the not insignificant matter of probation, which meant I had to be on my best behaviour for the whole of that first year. In a nutshell, I had to impress people to ensure my job was secure. Then there was the Southern Health Board contract that I'd signed, which obliged me to spend a certain number of hours in each of the three hospitals, adhering to a long list of obligations. And then there was the matter of ambition. As a returned emigrant, I was determined to bring home all the *nous* I'd acquired in fourteen years in exile. Even though I was again absurdly busy during my unexpected second mid-life internship, I was motivated by the huge appetite in all three hospitals for progress. So, I spun speedily around the city, creating three secretariats, three sets of departmental stationery (with a little red ambulance logo at the top), and invested as much time as I could in micromanagement and engagement with the managers.

Symbolically, I suppose, with Steve, my new consultant colleague, I set out *Ten Commandments in Emergency Medicine* for all staff, distilling the main concepts of modern emergency care, urging them above all to prioritise patients' distress and avoidable deterioration. My key organisational ambition was to convey to the nursing and medical staff the idea that much of the workload in the department was predictable, therefore it could be anticipated in our planning. In a nutshell, we knew roughly how many patients we were likely to see each day and if we were to draw an imaginary pyramid of emergency care, less than 5 per cent of patients at the top would need the Resuscitation Room, about 20 per cent would need a trolley (mainly because they were sick and elderly), and, at the bottom of the pyramid, roughly 75 per cent of our patients were ambulatory, meaning they walked in and out of the department on the same day. I also produced an infographic setting out the 'strategic steps to streamlining and improving the care of patients in Cork'.

In February 2000, these steps included a *Cork Emergency Medicine Forum* (a regular professional and social meeting for staff in Munster's emergency departments), audit, triage, teaching, review and good communication. Underpinning all of this good stuff, I put 'guiding principles, consensus and sound policy'. It all sounds so simple and straightforward now.

In practice, it was far from simple. I was scheduled to work in three separate emergency departments, in hospitals situated two miles, on average, from each other through city traffic, with separate staff and governance structures, and each with its own unique politics. On top of all that, each department was spectacularly under-resourced, in every sense, to deal with the roughly 100,000 patients coming through their collective portals. Still, I started as I meant to go on, enthusiastically shaking hands, meeting managers and new medical and nursing colleagues all around the city. I gradually acquired an office on all three sites and one secretary per department. There was the sainted and brilliant Terri Goulding, former secretary to the Director of Nursing at CUH, who had been shrewdly matched with me by the great Sheila Wall, doyenne of emergency nursing in Cork. There was the serenely unflappable Bernice O'Regan at the Mercy, and a shy but keen young Davina Hurst, just starting her career, at the South. All of these women 'minded' me fiercely from the outset.

In addition to Sheila, I made my usual beeline for the senior nurses in the three departments, like Mary Barry, Anne Hennessy, Norma O'Sullivan and Nuala Coughlan. As always, since that first day as an Intern, the nurses and the secretaries quickly became friends and indispensable allies and, with their support, I began to forge some sort of schedule that would allow me to rotate between the three emergency departments. I think there were two days each week when I wasn't travelling between the various hospitals, so I often swapped departments at lunchtime, and I tried to do just one scheduled Clinic a day, because each clinical (direct patient contact) minute tends to require a minute of writing notes or GP letters. The process is basically 'talk, touch, think, type …

repeat'. There was also a huge amount of non-clinical work to contend with. The letters poured in, to all three sites, inviting me to attend meetings, join committees, sit on interview panels for junior doctor appointments, approve release of notes to lawyers, and respond to complaints.

My first consideration in my efforts to improve and progress emergency care in the three hospitals was the nurses, and I listened carefully to them. They were clearly happy to have a new, even if 'part-time', consultant, as they saw it, but they were far from contented with the status quo in any of the departments. They summed it up simply: there wasn't enough space, senior cover, consensus on treatment, training for the non-consultant doctors, or nearly enough doctors.

And the mostly young medical trainees in the departments were – along with the patients – the group I was most worried about. For a start, as a former trainee I was all too aware of the needs and fears of graduates, and they'd long been my primary pastoral concern. I was conscious of the reliance of the health service on both sides of the Irish Sea on an erratic supply of graduates, which even twenty years ago was dwindling. And, as I got older, I'd come to really depend on the enthusiasm and infinitely varied talents of so many 'junior' doctors around me. Even then, I regularly quoted one of Colin Robertson's many wise thoughts uttered over lunch in the RIE: 'The only real legacy a doctor leaves is in the hearts and minds of the next generation'. Coming from one of the UK's most distinguished Professors of Emergency Medicine, and a truly great emergency physician, I elevated that notion to the level of evidence-based science.

Naturally, the non-consultant doctors were not exactly jumping for joy at the state of the emergency departments in Cork, where there was little consultant shopfloor presence to guide them, in the two city-centre departments at least, not to mention evidence-based policies, training or perceived support in-house. Nothing, however, distressed them as much as their rosters which, because there were so few of them, had them working flat out for long periods in congested and unsuitable units. Worst of all, in my view, they could not rely on guaranteed days off because they so often had to provide cover if one of their colleagues got sick.

In fact, of the ever-lengthening list of problems I compiled in those first months in Cork, the issue that infuriated me most, and symbolised the particular injustice faced by clinical staff in the city's emergency departments, was that of sick, special or study leave. I recall arriving in the South Infirmary one morning to find that its two-and-a-half emergency department rooms were stuffed with patients hoping to be seen or discharged, along with a packed waiting room, and finding that the single SHO (the senior house officer or first-year doctor) on duty for the morning had rung in sick. This meant that I was basically 'it'. I was the full complement of the staff available that morning, aside from the exhausted night-duty doctor, who was hoping to go home. So, while I pride myself on a rigorous courtesy, I was less than gruntled that morning after I rang the human resources department to tell them that the duty doctor was unable to work, and to seek their help. The response at the other end of the line was, 'Oh, hello, Dr Luke, actually what normally happens is that *you* ring around. Like, anyone you might know who's available, and ask them if they can do a shift for us. Is that okay?'

Now, even then I appreciated that I had just spent a decade in a huge UK hospital, with a huge emergency department, whose staffing problems were dealt with by a *staffing* department, but I admit that that was one of those moments when I realised that it was not just in terms of trauma and pre-hospital care that there were deficiencies in Ireland's health service. So, *mea culpa,* I allowed myself to be a little tetchy on the phone as I explained to my HR colleague that I was not *really* in a position to look after the numerous patients already in the department, in the waiting room, and outside my clinic room *and* to spend the next hour or two ringing around the city and county looking for replacement staff. That, I concluded, was properly the job of the *human resources* department, was it not? And sure enough, within an hour or so, as I got on with being just a doctor, the HR department found a temporary colleague for me.

One of the many problems of trying to run three separate departments simultaneously was the constant demands on my time, often leaving me unable to focus on what I wanted or needed to focus on. A pressing problem in this regard was how I was to run my Review Clinic. This was my exercise in monitoring the care of as many patients as possible, after I realised that some of the treatments being carried out in the department were far from ideal. Indeed, one orthopaedic surgeon used to berate me regularly about the quality of referrals to his Fracture Clinic from the city-centre departments which, in their defence, had been relatively consultant-less for years. He used to snort particularly at the 'Pavlovas' that were being applied to broken wrists when a proper plaster-of-Paris was required. Given my limited scheduled time in the city-centre departments, I aimed to address this issue by providing a safety-net review of patients within a day or two. This was partly for the benefit of the nursing staff, who periodically shook their heads at the management of some cases, but it was mainly for the benefit of the patients themselves. It seemed the least I could do to nibble into the huge caseload at the time.

The two smaller emergency departments were jointly seeing about 40,000 cases a year in 1999, so it was no mean feat to effect a step-change in quality. I thought the Review Clinics might offer a quick win in terms of morale, and they were an opportunity to get a sense of the caseload, to address the trainees' issues, and to teach. Above all, they were a chance to get to know the staff. The Clinics were hugely time-consuming, however, and before I knew it, I was seeing six, then ten, then up to twenty patients at each of them, as well as fresh cases that had suddenly 'gone off' (or suddenly deteriorated) on the shopfloor. Despite the enthusiastic assistance of the nursing and outpatient nursing staff, the Clinics often ran for two or three hours, or more. And then I usually had to scurry off to a committee meeting, tutorial or shopfloor session in one of my other hospitals. It was hamster-on-a-wheel stuff.

Aside from managing my hectic schedule, there were plenty of issues in Irish healthcare that seemed baffling and exasperating after my years abroad. One was the threatening 'legal letter', which used to arrive with a demand for a grovelling apology and compensation for someone's unacceptable wait or unhappiness with their care. As far as I could see, a few solicitors resorted routinely to these missives, and the hospitals sometimes seemed to capitulate to the demands immediately, without seriously investigating the complaint. Understandably, this reflected the 'absentee landlord' situation that characterised many Irish emergency departments in the 1990s, when there was no real consultant ownership of problems or – crucially – their solutions. In any case, after November 1999, I was quite robust in advising against further timidity on the part of the hospitals when it came to these letters. For one thing, I'd been trained by the NHS to recognise the 'educational value' of mistakes, so I was interested in examining every genuine error at length. Just as importantly, I knew all too well that legal or other complaints could be absolutely devastating for staff morale and for the reputation of a department. So my position was to stoutly defend the reputation of the service, as well as to carefully study and prevent future similar mistakes.

One initiative that was very helpful in improving patients' care was an extremely simple one: an information card for every patient. I introduced these in the three emergency departments, in early 2000, as a card on which was recorded quite clearly what was thought to be wrong with the patient, the name of the doctor who attended them in the ED, and the next step in their follow-up. Simple, but highly effective. I still think they were *one* neat solution to a multi-million-pound communication problem.

Another quirkily Irish phenomenon that upset me early on was the 'political phone call' coming through to a busy emergency department nursing station, from a local TD's office, sometimes via senior hospital management. CUH was where I most often encountered this, and the gist of the call was usually that someone's constituent was waiting on a trolley, or on a chair, and this was clearly a 'disgrace'. Self-evidently, it was implied, they needed to be admitted *immediately*. What was not so clear was how we were to explain to all the other patients waiting on trolleys or chairs that the patient who had just arrived (as far as the veterans of the corridor or waiting room were concerned) was to be admitted first, when the nurses were blue in the face apologising and explaining to all and sundry that there were *no* beds available in the wards, although 'as soon as there is, we'll get you up there'.

I like to think I never accommodated such a request. Aside from the discourtesy and the none-too-subtle bullying involved, it threatened to undermine completely the whole process of Triage, that systematic assessment of a patient's real urgency upon which a clinician's professional autonomy and authority rest. Worse than that, it represented the worst sort of parish-pump politics and fuelled an obvious injustice within the meritocracy of an emergency department, in which the severity of your illness determines your priority in any queue for care. Thankfully, this practice largely ended following sufficient adverse publicity.

It was one of my colleagues in Merseyside, John Bache, who in 1999 coined the elegant expression, 'medicine is an ecosystem with a wide diversity of habitats'. And I like to compare the emergency department with the foreshore of an Atlantic coastline, which is often submerged by high tides and is host to an enormous range of *human* species, and all sorts of flotsam and jetsam. It is an incredibly complex environment, subject to many meteorological, biological and geological influences, none of which is as tricky to manage as the human beings. I imagine this is the reality in every corner of the health service, whether in the community or the biggest hospital.

Or perhaps, like a Russian doll, to mix metaphors, the emergency department ecosystem is situated within and around larger and smaller systems. The outermost doll is, of course, the country itself, and in 1999 the major climatic change was the advent of the 'Celtic Tiger', a surge in the country's economic growth largely driven by foreign direct investment. This had transformed the common perception of Ireland as a quintessentially impoverished island to one characterised by remarkable prosperity, positivity and self-belief, at least in leafier parts of Dublin.

Another 'doll' is the political system across the island. In Northern Ireland, the new power-sharing Assembly was taking shape in late 1999 while, down south, a suddenly progressive Republic was headed by the country's second female president, Mary McAleese, and first female Tánaiste, Mary Harney. And it had a Finance Minister, Charlie McCreevy, famous for saying, 'If I have it, I'll spend it'. Such fiscal bonhomie seemed to be contagious and on 23 June 1999, in a letter to the *Irish Times*, the Minister for Health and Children, Brian Cowen, advertised his plans for a massive, well-funded overhaul of the infrastructure and staffing of pre-hospital care by ambulance professionals and GPs. Not before time, I remember thinking, but unsurprisingly the overhaul came 'dropping slow'.

Even if Ireland *is* a very small place, ultimately all politics comes down to the truly local, and the issues that were of concern to me included the emerging political dominance of CUH, which meant I often had to abandon my scheduled activities in the smaller hospitals to get back to Wilton for meetings to discuss the frequent twists and turns in CUH's strategic development. Then there was the impact of the relatively new Freedom of Information Act (FOI) on the healthcare system. In fact, FOI requests triggered the first minor dispute I recorded in my journal after I returned to

Ireland. This was with Denis Cusack, Professor in Forensic and Legal Medicine at UCD, who gave a very useful talk on FOI in early December 1999 at the South Infirmary. I remember taking issue with his analysis of the *implications* of FOI for hospitals, pointing out that the relatively innocuous Act was likely to pile yet more pressure on consultants, as they became obliged to vet large bundles of hospital records. These would all have to be signed off before being rapidly despatched to any lawyer requesting such paperwork under FOI legislation, with the threat of serious sanctions in the event of a delay.

Denis is a complete gentleman and a highly respected colleague, so I wrote to him afterwards to clarify any misunderstanding. I explained that a comparable growth in bureaucracy in the UK, under the rubric of 'accountability', had resulted in the medical profession being laid 'prostrate … on the rack', in the absence of extra time or assistance to process the increased paperwork. My simple plea was that the necessary resources be at least partly allocated. They weren't, of course. And over the following years, vetting paperwork for FOI requests became the predicted penitential exercise for all consultants in emergency medicine.

Shuttling between three hospitals was nothing short of madness, but it did give me a unique opportunity to contrast and compare the three units in detail. I was determined from the start to level the playing field between the various emergency departments in Cork, and in Tralee across the border in County Kerry. And I insisted that the provision of emergency healthcare in the city and counties should mean 'a single service on multiple sites'. Naively idealistic to a fault, I argued that the quality of care for patients should be the same, 'regardless of the portal of entry'. I couldn't see any reason why treatment of acute illness or injury should depend on where a patient was randomly directed or delivered by ambulance. Not only that, despite my previous youthful enthusiasm for 'bigger, brighter, better' (after working in an enormous emergency department in Liverpool), I was now convinced that there should be a ceiling in terms of a department's caseload. Perhaps naively, again, I started to suggest that no department should really be dealing with more than, say, 60,000 new patients per annum.

Of course, by 1999, CUH, which had the major emergency department in the south of Ireland, was seeing over 50,000 cases annually, and as with every department in these islands, there seemed to be an inbuilt inflation of about 4 per cent per annum in term of the number of attendances. The entries in my journals in early 2000 remind me painfully that the greatest difficulty in that first year, and for years afterwards, related to adult and adolescent patients needing psychological or psychiatric support. This meant that while they were 'directed' to the ED, they often ended up waiting there for hours, or even days, to be admitted to suitable facilities which then, as now, were in short supply. That included adolescents who were clearly in crisis, who had repeatedly presented in the previous weeks with deliberate self-harm (like cutting or overdose), or people with cannabis-related psychosis or alcohol withdrawal who were recovering slowly but needed to be physically more-or-less asymptomatic before they could be accommodated in a psychiatric unit bed.

My first year in Cork ended in late November 2000 when my probation period was concluded. I'd done enough to secure my place, and my full contract with the Health Board was confirmed. In a sense, I had been on my best behaviour for the duration and I only began to feel professionally free when the contract was assured. But, privately, I spent years after my arrival in Cork ruminating about my decision to take on such a crazily demanding job. Not a day went by without a fresh crisis in one, or all, of the hospitals and, by January 2000, I expected phone calls every day from HR or ED staff looking for miracle solutions to intractable problems. Easily the most troubling difficulty was in recruiting enough doctors to staff the three departments. This undoubtedly reflected the great unhappiness among most junior nursing and medical staff across the country in that first year back, with industrial action by nurses in November 1999 and rallies held by doctors in many hospitals, protesting against their 100-hour weeks. I have vivid memories of the photographs in the *Irish Examiner* of placard-waving nurses outside the Mercy and CUH, as well as reports of the de facto leader of the non-consultant doctors, Mick Molloy, a future President of the IMO and consultant in emergency medicine, standing on a canteen chair in CUH addressing his comrades like a 21st-century Jim Larkin.

I was reminded that I too had attended rallies in the early 1980s in Dublin about trainees' conditions. But, oddly, something that never occurred to me while I was in exile was that the working conditions for Irish medical trainees, and the brutally long shifts they had to work, would *not* have been fixed after I left in 1986. This was despite the fact that all over the world, from Europe to North America, limits on doctors' hours had been introduced because of clear evidence that exhaustion was harmful not just to the medics but sometimes lethally so for their patients. In fact, as far back as the mid-

1980s, I remember reading about the notorious case of Libby Zion, a 19-year-old patient in a New York hospital, who was found to have died as a direct result of the fatigue and inadequate support of a grossly overworked medical trainee.

This scandalised enough people, there at least, to see regulations introduced in the USA restricting junior medics' hours to about 80 per week and requiring senior medical staff to be present far more often in hospitals out-of-hours. I was highly supportive of the non-consultant doctors' grievance, but as a consultant I also had to worry about not harming patients. And I suppose I am of a generation of medics who'd find it next to impossible to go out on strike, myself.

Sadly, within weeks of arriving back in Ireland, I was finding the demands of the work on three sites, the commuting and the political challenges in each institution absolutely exhausting, and frankly I was finding it difficult to cope. My long-suffering wife recently reminded me that I was actually seriously floundering and, in the summer of 2000, I admitted to her that I'd made 'a terrible mistake' in taking the job. Thinking back now, I recall the terrible dread and sickness I used to feel in my stomach every time I drove to CUH, from our rented house in Frankfield. This was a short distance from the Kinsale Road roundabout as the crow flies, but a good twenty minutes as the traffic then flowed. I remember how the nightmarish roundabout, the design of which *caused* countless accidents as well as traffic mayhem, seemed typical of the way the country was run, and perhaps the health service too. At night, lying in bed, unable to sleep, I was racked with anguish about my decision to sign a contract that was described as 'ludicrous', 'insane' and 'impossible' by many of my friends and colleagues, new and old.

It was a happy coincidence, then, that one of them, Ann Payne, the hugely enthusiastic Registrar at the Mercy, was also a psychiatrist, who provided more than a little cheerful counselling for me on our tea breaks. This was just as well, as by then I'd started to have regular palpitations as well as insomnia. Victoria recalled how one night, instead of just lying there awake, I'd suddenly leapt out of bed and scribbled my last will and testament, making some bizarre bequests to friends and former colleagues.

The fundamental problem was that all three departments were permanently bursting at the seams, with shortages of space, staff and essential support, so I was fighting a losing battle in all of them at the same time. Worse still than the workload and incessant driving between hospitals, I'd begun to dread interaction with certain colleagues. Two or three in each hospital seemed to thrive on being unhelpful, and one or two seemed to enjoy baiting or bullying me, and while I'd been used to dealing with a few difficult individuals in the huge consultant cohort at the Royal, this was usually sorted over a few pints on a Friday night. However, I was unable to properly socialise with enough of my new consultant colleagues in Cork due to the sheer busyness of the job, my incessant movement, and the fact that I didn't really know where to start.

The result was that small, avoidable humiliations coalesced for me across the city, at the same time as I found myself frustrated for weeks without a printer in CUH, or an office in the South Infirmary, or operating from a tiny, windowless storeroom at the back of the Mercy emergency department, politely accommodating the perceived slights, manipulation or indifference of a few colleagues. It didn't help for me to think of the enormous upstairs office I'd enjoyed all to myself in the Royal. Even if the shopfloor there was always chaotic and congested, I could get away now and again to engage in a telephone or face-to-face conversation in peace, in a proper office above the fray, and get some correspondence, staff interaction or administrative work done. And while I know it would make pretty dull TV, the one glaring omission in every TV or movie depiction of emergency room life, no matter how otherwise exciting or sexy, is the vast amount of bureaucratic activity required of all doctors and nurses, as well as the secretarial and clerical staff. Along with a lot of patient contact, correspondence and written proposals arrived in sackloads for me at each ED. Sometimes these seemed innocuous, but they had long-term ramifications, like the development of heart attack protocols or the surge in psychiatric attendances we were asked to accommodate in the Mercy in early 2000.

Looking back at my journal, I'm struck by the way three of the biggest extracurricular projects of my first half-decade back in Ireland were put to me before the end of my probationary year. By then I'd already been invited by Garda Superintendent Kieran McGann to give a talk on 'nightclub medicine' to an assembly of senior Gardaí and publicans from Cork city and county. And remarkably, this evolved quite quickly, with the energetic support of the Assistant Commissioner, into 'Club Cork', a joint HSE/Garda/National Ambulance Service programme of on-site training for all staff in the biggest clubs and pubs in the southern capital in relation to alcohol and drug misuse and its complications. I know that for several years all the partners in the exercise, myself included, were extremely enthusiastic about its impact.

Then there was the *Initial Management of the Severely Injured Patient*, a project commissioned by the Clinical Guidelines Committee of the Royal College of Surgeons of Ireland. Or, I should say, its chairman, my erstwhile hero, Professor Niall O'Higgins. Its aim was to set out the needs for and outline of a national trauma system to deal with the most seriously injured patients in the country and to devise a series of evidence-based clinical pathways, or algorithms, for their initial management. This slowly became a weighty but elegant 68-page document, published in 2003, with a lot of work by yours truly and another future surgical star, Ronan Cahill.

During this time, I also received an invitation from the Chief Executive Officer of CUH, Tony McNamara, to help sort out the problems the hospital was having with its Interns. These first-year medical graduates had been expressing unhappiness with the quality of their training in the final years of medical school in UCC, as well as their actual experiences in their twelve months on the wards (like most of their counterparts nationally). As a former medical educationalist in Liverpool, who'd led the delivery of a new Education Centre at the Royal, it was a subject close to my heart. So despite the illogicality of a floundering physician taking on yet more work, I abruptly found myself with a fourth job, as Intern Tutor and Director of Postgraduate Medical Education at CUH, in charge of an as-yet-non-existent postgraduate medical education service.

As a result of this new string to my bow, I set up a new clinical skills course in the summer of 2001, at the behest of Professor Eamonn Quigley, the Head of the Medical School. This two-day Final MB Clinical Skills Course aimed to address the deficiencies in practical training identified by the medical graduates. It involved a series of 'stations' scattered about the Boole Library, Anatomy Department and Mini-Restaurant on the often sun-soaked UCC campus, at which I had assigned some of the best clinical teachers I could find in Cork. There they taught the 100 or so MB (or Bachelor of Medicine) graduates the practicalities of prescribing drugs, inserting urinary catheters or intravenous cannulae, basic life support and defibrillation. Some of the newly minted doctors were learning these skills for the first time, just a week or two before they started on the wards, so they were both keen and grateful for the teaching. That was encouraging, given that the course was a massive logistical exercise, which was followed up with a specific induction course in CUH and the other UCC hospitals.

The secret to our success was undoubtedly the willingness of so many medical and nursing colleagues to give their time and energy, the support of UCC staff like Tomas Tyner, not to mention the ever-encouraging Professor Quigley, and the sheer brilliance and heroic input of Terri Goulding, who moved from her secretarial position with me in the emergency department at CUH, to effectively running – and *being* – the postgraduate medical education service at CUH. Happily, the course was a huge hit with the university, the graduates and their parents, and it got honourable mentions in the pages of the *Irish Times* and the *Irish Examiner*.

At the end of each year's course, I asked the Interns who were about to finish to offer their 'Seven Habits of Highly Effective Interns' to their successors. Some of the tips I used repeatedly over the following few years came from a particularly impressive Intern at CUH, Conor Deasy. His recommended habits included, 'Be enthusiastic and kind-hearted, play it safe, take deep breaths in the x-ray department, take a serious temperature seriously, and consult people you admire about your career.'

I remember thinking at the time how much his ideas resonated with those of Professor O'Higgins, twenty years previously, as well as my own. And it occurred to me that, while the means of delivering medical care may change constantly, really great doctors know from the outset that the basics of excellent patient care *always* remain the same: (1) kindness, (2) enthusiasm and (3) good humour. Moreover, as the years went by and I toiled in the city's emergency departments, I would think of the fun and the satisfaction I felt each June when the Final MB Clinical Skills Course was in full swing around the half-empty UCC campus, with teachers and young graduates alike laughing and bursting with enthusiasm. And I would conclude again and again that the very best part of medicine is when younger and older medics are learning from one another, and enjoying each other's company. Over the next 15 years, I would have many of these moments – but I would also find myself faced with some of the worst aspects of medicine and the relationships between its practitioners.

Patients … and Patience

T he aspect of a visit to an Irish emergency department that patients probably find hardest to deal with is the inevitable delay in getting in, getting out and getting answers. If you're lucky, you could be in and out within an hour or two. But even that commonest of questions posed by patients and anxious companions, 'So, what's wrong?', can be hard to answer. At least, at the time it is first asked. My standard approach to this kind of query, and I'm not being entirely facetious, is to say (to students at least), 'I'll tell you exactly what's wrong with this patient in six weeks.' And even that is a qualified truth because while 'mysteries do unfold', as the song goes, there are times when neither a lengthy stay in hospital nor an autopsy yields the precise cause of a patient's condition. Still, *time will tell* is as important a mantra at the frontline as any ABC of first-aid intervention.

Now, before you shout, 'Where's the senior decision-maker?!', as politicians call us consultants, I should explain about the *limitations* of consultants. I believe that the palm of my hand and the tip of my thumb are pretty effective at identifying injury, infection and inflammation, as a direct result of examining thousands of patients. My *gestalt*, or diagnostic hunch, about patients' injuries or ailments is reasonably impressive too, for the same reason, but the problem is that both are spread very thin. It is a fact that there are relatively few consultants in my speciality in Ireland. I think there were a dozen or so when I returned from the UK in 1999, and there are still only around 75 in the country's 35-odd public and private emergency departments, which cater for over 1.2 million attendances annually. For most of my twenty years' frontline clinical practice in Cork, there were over 120,000 patients attending five urgent care facilities between the city, Mallow and Bantry annually, but just five or six consultants, most of whom had competing multi-site commitments, like me. What that meant in practice, and what it still means, is that there are simply too few consultants in most EDs to see cases around-the-clock.

And of course the scans, x-rays, myriad tests and even the consultants' eyes and hands are only part of the answer to what is wrong with every patient. In practice, time alone reveals what's going on with most cases, and the application of time is often the most important diagnostic test of all. That is why admitting a patient for a few hours or days to the clinical decision unit (CDU) or observation ward of an ED may be the most realistic way to predict the path of recovery, or to establish an otherwise uncertain diagnosis. As I said before, most issues *crystallise* or *dematerialise* in the CDU. In other words, most minor injuries or mild illnesses subside with a little TLC, time and careful nursing, but a few significant – sometimes fatal – diagnoses only become manifest over a period of hours.

Obviously, getting one of those rare senior emergency physicians or Advanced Nurse Practitioners to review a patient's progress within hours of their first presentation is not only common sense and a better use of a scarce human resource, it is invaluable for patient satisfaction, risk management and quality assurance. It also provides a great opportunity to teach students about the diagnosis, treatment and trajectory of many injuries and ailments.

The way that multiple injuries reveal themselves is a good example of *unfolding mysteries*. Take the middle-aged male who feels 'quite capable of sorting out the gutters' himself, ascends a wobbly ladder and in a matter of nanoseconds finds himself lying in pain on the gravel below. The resulting injuries can be severe, but provided the poor man hasn't sustained a devastating head or spinal injury, the first thing to do is *not panic*, but to remember the 'compassion equation' – empathy plus action – and get on with relieving his distress.

In Cork, this scenario typically involves a concerned partner who's phoned the ambulance from the house, and a concussed or distressed patient who may need snug spinal immobilisation and oral, inhaled or injected pain relief en route to the Resus Room at CUH. There, a team will assess him systematically, looking for brain injury, spinal cord damage or collapsed lung and so on. In a matter of minutes, the casualty may have drips coming out of his arms, ECG leads draped over his chest, and a series of quickfire x-rays where he lies, before being transferred to the main x-ray department for a CT brain scan, or a 'pan-scan', in which the brain and torso are scanned, from neck to hip, to screen for organ damage, bleeding into cavities or broken bones. Then, once the serious stuff has been excluded, the patient may be transferred to the observation ward or CDU to recuperate. And there, the following day, having recovered under the watchful eye and tender mercies of an experienced senior emergency nurse, the consultant may find the victim chatty and relieved to be alive, but still 'not really able to walk'. And, in short order, a fracture of the talus or tibial plateau, those parts at the middle of his ankle or knee, may sometimes be spotted, even though there was no mention whatsoever of a sore ankle or knee in the ambulance or Resus Room notes of the evening before.

The explanation for such 'missed' diagnoses lies in the realms of human psychology and physiology. In a nutshell, 'bigger injuries distract from little injuries', so a head injury with 'concussion' (i.e. nothing abnormal on the brain scan) will cause a lot more initial concern than a normal-looking ankle or knee, especially when the victim is complaining of a headache or a sore ribcage.

And it is only the next morning, as the rib pain and head injury symptoms (brain fog and banging headache) subside, that the pain of the lower limb injury starts to make itself felt. Moreover, the bleeding associated with a bruise or broken bone takes time to stretch the surrounding tissues and to excite inflammation which, in its own good time, creates the swelling, redness and tenderness that are so obvious on the ward round. The same sort of potentially tricky situation occurs in lots of injuries, like bone bruises, hairline fractures of the scaphoid wrist bone or rib fractures, all of which are mostly associated with normal x-rays at first. The good news is that such injuries settle naturally of their own accord, and the medic's role is mainly to support this process and reassure the patient. But it can be hard to explain to people afterwards why a fracture was not spotted immediately. The answer to that important question is, yet again, *experience* and *time*.

Evidence from hospital emergency departments world-wide over the last hundred years has shown that every injury is unique, but there tends to be patterns in the way they evolve, become visible clinically or on x-ray, and then settle. For instance, the scaphoid bone, one of eight carpal bones in a sort of Rubik's cube arrangement in the wrist, is a particularly devious fracture. That is why a second x-ray is so often required ten days after an initial injury to the bone, or a scan even sooner, if available. We know this primarily as in the past we kept missing broken scaphoids, because the bone often looks quite 'normal' on the first x-ray. Then as the fracture site slowly bleeds, hydraulic pressure rises, the fragments gradually drift apart, and the break becomes obvious when the second x-ray is done routinely a week or so later (or a year later when the patient represents due to their still-painful wrist). So the trick in emergency care is to accumulate enough experience to have a decent hunch that a particular injury exists, and to treat the patient accordingly.

The consequence is that the older emergency physician's diagnostic radar is always on, not least because of bitter experience. And this applies especially in the pressurised environment of the emergency department, where you learn over time that *assumption* is the mother of all mistakes. It's not that you can't rely on the previous doctor to have come to the correct conclusions about the patient in front of you now, it's just that you *mustn't rely* on them. Every case requires a fresh pair of eyes, and a completely open mind, otherwise a dangerous diagnostic bias called 'anchoring' may come into play. This is one of the commonest hazards in a busy ED, and it is a source of many lawsuits.

What it means in practice is that, when a series of healthcare professionals (doctors, nurses, radiographers, physiotherapists) encounter a patient in the hospital setting, they are usually under pressure, so they may take at face value – or become *fixated* on – the working diagnosis of the first of their colleagues to see the patient. Often this is a Triage nurse, who is generally the first to meet most patients, and whose objective is to quickly assess the urgency of each case, using a limited amount of information (say, a GP letter or the patient's main symptoms) and measurements of vital signs (blood pressure, heart rate, temperature and so on). This is done to avoid the first-come-first-served approach of yore, which led to the politest patients dying in waiting rooms as they were bumped back by noisy queue-jumpers.

The Triage nurse's note might say '*? Tension Headache*' as the primary issue, and there may be nothing else noteworthy in their quick preliminary assessment. Anchoring is what can then occur when each subsequent doctor or nurse meets the patient and, in going through their clinical notes, sees the phrase '*? Tension Headache*' under Complaint and begins to assume that is the *actual* diagnosis. In other words, they remain anchored to the first diagnostic idea. The young patient concerned may go on to have all sorts of blood tests and a brain scan as the headache persists throughout the hours he waits to be assessed, reassessed and admitted to the CDU. He may even be scheduled for a lumbar puncture to tap and test the liquid about his spinal cord for evidence of meningitis. Hopefully, the patient will be seen during the ward round by a consultant or other senior emergency physician. And the latter may not be really convinced that there is anything going on with the brain, in the absence of confusion, neck or head pain on straining, or impaired vision. Instead, the doctor recognises an exhausted undergraduate who is facing into their final exams and has been burning the candle at both ends, studying and working part-time in a local petrol station. The chances are that all the tests will be normal, or at most marginally out of kilter. Why? Because rare diseases are rare. If you look out your window now, the bird flying past is more likely to be a sparrow than a golden eagle.

Thus a brain tumour is highly unlikely. And, when further enquires are made, it becomes clear that the young patient's main complaints are severe fatigue, a niggling cough that he forgot to mention, and a banging frontal headache. There really is nothing more to find, although the patient's temperature has risen since he met the Triage nurse and is now hovering at the top of the normal range. And listening to his chest with a stethoscope reveals some scratchy or crackly noises just below the right shoulder blade. It then takes a chest x-ray, not a brain scan, to confirm that it is a relatively simple pneumonia that is causing the headache and loss of energy, which is overlapping with his exhaustion.

The point about anchoring is that disease and diagnosis are both constantly evolving, dynamic processes, so *signs* (what we see) and *symptoms* (what we feel) can all change between the first encounter in an ED and the next, especially if a few hours elapse in between. But still, even the most experienced doctors will encounter conditions they've never seen before.

One of the best-known examples of an 'evolving' case that I've seen was that of the 24-year-old actor Conor Madden, which achieved worldwide coverage in 2011. He was playing the lead role in Shakespeare's *Hamlet* on the Everyman Theatre stage in Cork, and in the sword-fight scene at the climax of the play, his mortal enemy, Laertes, is supposed to stab him with a poison-tipped sword. Unfortunately, on this occasion the actor's face was *actually* pierced with a round-tipped replica rapier. The next day's *Irish Times* commented, 'You can't have Hamlet without the prince', and recounted how the sword-fighting accident had cut short the production. However, the play's director reassured the reporter: 'Conor is fine. It's quite a complex sword-fight and I'm amazed it doesn't happen more. It was just one of those rare occasions. The sword caught him under the eye, and he pulled back to avoid it but got a small cut. I think he went into a bit of shock.' The reporter added that the patient was to resume playing the role of the Prince of Denmark after skipping just a couple of performances.

However, Mr Madden was readmitted to CUH over the next few days, and his condition was far from fine. In fact, within weeks he was confined to a wheelchair, unable to feed or shower himself and had difficulty moving, speaking or seeing clearly. What initially looked like a nick in the skin below his eye turned out to have been like a deep stiletto wound, which caused an injury to his nervous system that unfolded slowly over the following few days. In some respects, it was like a small calibre bullet wound, with a deceptively unimpressive surface appearance, but severe damage beneath. And, unfortunately, according to reports on the BBC World Service and many newspapers, it took the remarkably brave and determined Conor Madden years to recover after that final fateful scene at the Everyman.

Another case that was widely reported in the Irish media was even rarer than a theatrical sword-fight injury, and this was a case which involved my old friend and colleague, Steve (now Professor) Cusack. He had come into work at CUH early one morning, as was his habit, and had gone into his office at around 6.30 a.m. to collect his thoughts before the first meeting of the day. He noticed a distinct whiff of cigarette smoke in the air but thought no more of it and headed off to do his CDU ward round. During the round, he was informed that a patient with a severe headache who was due to have a spinal tap or lumbar puncture had 'disappeared' off the ward.

This was not an unusual thing to hear as patients frequently take their own discharge from various parts of every ED, so Steve carried on seeing the rest of the patients in the CDU before heading back to his office. It was only as he sat at his desk, and looked down at his feet, that he discovered, curled up under his desk, the body of the missing patient. It transpired that the poor man had taken a lethal overdose of medication that he had himself brought into the hospital. He was actually recorded on CCTV footage in a public part of the department 'taking a lot of pills' in the small hours of the night, and an autopsy revealed that the amount of synthetic opioid taken was such that, even if he'd been found sooner, the outcome was unlikely to have been altered. Tellingly, no cause was found for the original headache.

It was a dreadful story, and the city coroner made a point, during her subsequent inquest, of suggesting that every patient admitted to hospital should be asked what medication they had brought with them, if any. This was a sensible idea, and one of the more grimly consistent themes of a life in medicine is that lessons are mostly learned from mistakes and mishaps.

Having said that, I wish one other important lesson could be learned, and that is that doctors – even hospital consultants – are human beings. I was genuinely shocked by the way Steve was treated after he made the terrible finding that morning in his office. What Steve needed at the very least was time out and a few kind words. But it *seemed* that the only thing that mattered to some people was that the relevant paperwork was completed, not that a member of staff involved might have been severely traumatised by the events. I've known Steve since we were teenagers, and he is one of the most stoic medics I know, but just because older emergency physicians have a self-evident pedigree of resilience, it cannot be assumed that they are made of stone. I'm pretty sure that few other people would have been so cool, calm and collected after such a tragedy. And while Steve and I have very similar value systems, there's probably one key difference between him and me. I would have been profoundly angered by the lack of sympathy shown afterwards. Then again, many of us who work within the healthcare system are only too aware that it often seems to be the opposite of caring towards its own employees. And I am not referring to the 'mission statements' of many institutions, which are full of the most trite, cringe-inducing nonsense to be found on headed stationery anywhere. I'm talking about *people* with little capacity for empathy.

Clearly, it would be wrong to imply that the sort of cases admitted under the care of the emergency medicine consultants at CUH are always dramatic or disastrous, but there is nearly always some kind of drama involved when it comes to weird or wonderful diagnoses.

The most dramatic sort of presentation – where there is often no discernible medical cause – is probably a 'pseudoseizure', with bizarre thrashing movements quite unlike those of a typical seizure. Next comes 'pseudocoma', which mainly requires time, careful observation and experience to identify, plus the careful tickling of eyelashes. Only the genuinely unconscious can avoid blinking in response to this. These issues fall under the heading of 'functional neurological disorders', mysterious issues of the brain circuits rather than the anatomy, which is usually normal on scans. One day, I expect we'll understand – and treat – them a great deal better.

And there are always plenty of colourful sources of avoidable worry on a CDU. 'Sexual' headaches are a good example. Obviously, there is the *Not tonight, darling* type, but others can be a feature of an intra-uterine contraceptive coil or a contraceptive bar inserted in the patient's arm. And the most spectacular, mostly male, version is the sudden 'celphalgia', or startlingly severe headache resulting in *coitus interruptus*, which is frightening but benign. This often-embarrassing condition is said to affect as many as 1 per cent of the population (or at least that number come to hospital) and is reported to be associated with kneeling, overexcitement (a conundrum in the context), and the use of certain drugs like cannabis, amphetamine and sildenafil, a medication used for erectile dysfunction. It is also one of the conditions which no medical graduate ever seems to recognise. Even in 2021, it seems, 'sex, drugs and rock'n'roll' remain excluded from the medical curriculum.

Management of these comes under the heading of crystallise or dematerialise, so time is needed to observe and figure such cases out, as well as a little telepathy between medical and nursing staff. One of the highlights of my twenty years working at CUH was conducting CDU rounds with

Anna Dillon, the wonderful nurse in charge. Anna could transmit a crucial judgement and an unerring sense of something being amiss with the merest twitch of her mouth, or a certain upward dart of her eyes, as she pulled the cubicle curtains across. Her brand of moral and intellectual assistance made for highly enjoyable and efficient ward rounds. Moreover, it could get personal. I remember the dismay I felt when I received notice of the first and only complaint about me to the Medical Council in nearly 40 years of practice. The allegations were vague in the extreme, and even the object of the complaint seemed to be uncertain, insofar as a long list of doctors were named as having been 'very rude' to the complainant on a CDU round, and it was only as, one after another, each name was excluded that mine came up. In any event, it turned out that the complainant was not *compos mentis*, and the complaint was dismissed. But Steve and Anna both testified that they'd 'never met a more polite and kindly doctor' than yours truly, and the supposed incident was so 'out of character' as to be simply not credible.

I was extremely grateful to both of them for their support in my hour of need, and thankfully the Council found that there was no *prima facie* case, and the complaint was dismissed. It may be hard for non-medics to appreciate the stress that such a grievance can cause, even when it is unfounded. But the conditions in which we have worked have been so awful for so long that I find it easy to imagine how this sort of complaint could prove a final straw for a worn-out medic in an emergency department. It is one of the reasons I sometimes take on Medical Council-related advisory work, because I can think of few other aspects of a doctor's life in which the truth matters quite so much and where injustice *must* be prevented.

All these cases remind me that when it comes to a packed emergency department Resus Room, Cubicle, Review Clinic, or CDU, there is simply no substitute for experience. First of all, in terms of putting oneself in the shoes of a patient *or* another colleague and providing that sometimes vital support. And second, getting back to the bigger picture, *diagnostically*, because a magic wand, like an ultrasound probe, may not always be available and a fancy scan simply cannot be deployed for every case. Such an approach would quickly overwhelm every hospital radiology department and would bankrupt the whole institution, too. In short, experience will always be crucial in ensuring the creaking ship sails as smoothly as possible, in the circumstances. And this requires patience on the part of everybody concerned.

Speaking of experience, the CDU in Cork University Hospital accommodates hundreds of patients annually, and the vast majority are successfully managed there, without needing onward referral. It has provided invaluable opportunities to scrutinise common and important treatment regimes, like those needed to treat patients with asthma, allergy, surface infections, head injury, overdoses, collapsed lung, or alcohol withdrawal syndrome (the DTs or *delirium tremens*, as it is known). And it has enabled us to pilot professional interventions, such as those by Alcohol Specialist Nurses, (Psychosocial) Crisis Nurses, or Inclusion Health Specialist Nurses. The differences such systematic improvements in care and specialist nurse involvement have made to our patients have been remarkable, if not historic, in my view. And their involvement is based on yet another lesson that has been learned in emergency healthcare over the past 50 years or more. This is the realisation that there is usually a brief window of opportunity in patients' lives that is ideal for a so-called *brief intervention*. This is typically 'the morning after the night before', in the CDU, when the effects of alcohol, drugs and anger have worn off, and a 'teachable moment' presents itself. Just between semi-coma and desperate hangover, there may be a sense of remorse on the part of the patient when they realise that something must be done about their habits or inclinations.

Mostly, it involves people on their umpteenth visit, or those threatened with the breakdown of relationships with the people they love the most. But that's okay. All it takes is a few minutes' conversation.

And here, I should add, that my greatest hope for emergency medicine in the next 20 years is not just that we become ever better at resuscitating the critically ill and injured, or processing the walking wounded ever-more efficiently. I am certain that huge progress is already being made in those respects. What I really hope is that, as we deal compassionately and effectively with patients, we also recognise the main reasons why they become chronically and acutely ill or injured: the anxiety, loneliness or buried grief which drive people to over-consume sugar, tobacco and a myriad of stress-relieving intoxicants. I hope that we recognise that most people in the emergency department are actually there by choice: not always in the sense of 'I fancy a trip to the ED today', but in terms of the culmination of years of overdoing the sugar, salt, tobacco, alcohol or recreational drugs and so on.

This all means that, in 2021, we don't just treat the wound, the bruise or the overdose – we try to treat the underlying history, context and adverse childhood experiences, or rather the consequences of such experiences. After all, every older emergency physician and nurse recognises that the greatest self-harmers, those who have the worst so-called 'personality disorder' or impulsive behaviour, are often the ones upon whom the most grotesque emotional, physical or sexual harm was visited when they were children. This is why I keep saying, *Difficulty makes people difficult*. Really and truly.

It also explains why I believe that one of the greatest developments in emergency medicine and nursing in my lifetime has been the appointment of specialist nurses to which I've referred, and Liaison Psychiatrists, the sort who specialise in the interface between emergency medicine and Psychiatry. This means that we can now effectively *resuscitate* the victims of self-harm or anger; we can allow them to *recover* safely and securely as inpatients; and, as they prepare to recover outside the hospital, we can offer the possibility of a *long-term solution*. Or the beginnings of such. So nowadays, the Crisis Nurse can screen for addictive or self-harming tendencies, the Inclusion Health Nurse can arrange accommodation and outreach services, and the Alcohol Liaison Nurse can connect a newly willing and recovering patient with inpatient or outpatient services. These specialist nurses can also arrange referral to an enormous range of psychiatric, public health and social services.

I am not suggesting for once that high-tech medicine and nursing combined with expertise and compassion can sort everybody. But what I am saying is that we are making real progress towards a situation where we can at least *offer* this kind of holistic approach to most of the people who attend an emergency department in Ireland. And for those who worry about the rise and rise of artificial intelligence, I would remind them that it will always be brilliant nurses and doctors, not marvellous technology, who work the real miracles in all of our emergency departments.

In terms of the bigger picture, I hope that honest public debate in this country may also allow us to admit that many people do in fact say to themselves: 'The best thing for my ingrowing toe-nail/chronic skin disorder/long-term pain problem or whatever is to head to the emergency department because although I may have to wait for hours, once I'm registered there is a decent chance that I will be plugged into the system and I will eventually get to see the relevant specialist much sooner than I otherwise would.' Only when we realise that this is happening, and stop wasting time with semantics or mudslinging, will we be able to either allocate the necessary resources or create better alternatives to such visits to our EDs.

And I hope that politicians and policymakers start to recognise that healthcare in the emergency department has become exponentially more complex, due to globalisation, our extended lifespan and people's expectations. Moreover, technological possibilities also mean that what can – and must – be done before patients get to a hospital ward is ever-more challenging, from understanding dozens of patient languages to the technicalities of non-invasive ventilation for the breathless elderly and those with COVID-19, from the logistics of getting heart attack cases to a regional cardiac catheter lab to the vigilance required to contain exotic infections or resurgent TB, life is far more convoluted in the ED than it was even a decade ago.

Above all, I hope that there will be a greater awareness among healthcare professionals, patient associations and politicians that when an ED gets really crowded, *everyone* within it may become angry and frightened and sometimes a little less cooperative or able to concentrate. This is the reality which everyone must address urgently. Because, sadly, the greatest obstacle to near-miracles in emergency departments is not really a want of technology or indeed vision but the challenge of *professional burnout*, a distressing dis-ease that results largely from the oppressive atmosphere which so often develops these days within emergency departments, and from which we must protect our most precious assets – the medical and nursing staff who are not just there for one or two days but for years at a time.

The Magic of Medicine

'I'm sorry, but I seem to have left my magic wand at home...' used to be a standard sarcastic quip among weary nurses and doctors in emergency departments when faced with particularly difficult people or situations. Nowadays, of course, many medics in these departments *do* actually use semi-magical wands, called ultrasound probes, in their daily work to look for foreign bodies in the soft tissues of a foot, a collapsed lung in someone with chest pain, or for heart movement during a cardiac arrest. Many even use the probes routinely to put lines into veins or arteries.

In fact, there's now an abundance of technology in healthcare everywhere in Ireland and the UK. There was a time when that meant a blood pressure cuff, or sphygmomanometer, a glass thermometer and an ECG monitor. So in your typical emergency department, in 2021, you can expect to have your temperature measured in a few seconds with a probe inserted into your ear, your arterial oxygen levels calculated by a probe clipped onto your finger for 20 seconds, not to mention the shape and rate of your heartbeat, the identity of toxicological agents in your urine, or the levels of sodium, chloride, potassium, pH, bicarbonate and carbon dioxide in your blood in a matter of minutes.

Add the x-ray facilities and CT scanners that are now present in many departments, as well as anaesthetic equipment for supporting the very sick, and it really is remarkable how advanced the diagnostic capacity is at the front door of even small hospitals. It means that emergency department staff can get a remarkable insight into the function of most of a patient's organs within an hour or so of their arrival.

There's a mesmerising array of advanced technology elsewhere in hospital laboratories, pathology and imaging departments. Other science-fiction-come-true developments mean that medical students and postgraduate trainees now learn many of the proficiencies they need for trauma and emergency care in simulation labs, like the ASSERT unit in UCC. These facilities have largely taken over from the *moulage* or 'pretend' scenarios of just a decade ago, which used relatively primitive manikins and anatomical models. These days, learning skills can be like playing video games, or using virtual reality sets. Such simulation would certainly have been described as magical by previous generations and is so popular that teams from the country's medical schools compete to get the best SIM scenario outcomes in annual competitions.

And, yet, I still believe that there is another kind of magic involved in medicine, especially the kind practised at 'the pointy end'. This magic is also called instinct, and is something I acquired through observation, imitation and practice in busy emergency departments in Dublin, Edinburgh, Liverpool and Cork. I worry occasionally that the conjuring tricks of technology are sometimes prized above the old-fashioned wizardry of my medical youth. Mind you, both kinds of magic need a lot of practice, and imagination.

My limited capacity to concentrate thwarted me for years as a medical student, until the penny dropped, and I realised that the real source of a physician's diagnostic skills lay in studying his *patients,* not his books. The fact is that becoming a good doctor is fundamentally a matter of carefully observing and listening to enough patients. I'd suggest 10,000 of them for a start. That's the figure famously cited by Malcolm Gladwell in his 2008 bestseller, *Outliers,* when he set out his notion that the key to becoming an expert at *anything* was 10,000 hours' practice at one's craft, be it singing, playing a cello, or tinkering with a computer. The number was based on a slightly flawed study of violinists, but I still like the idea that – combined with talent and opportunity – the number of patients a doctor treats largely determines his or her competence.

I reckon I've treated over 125,000 patients in my time in emergency departments and I've read countless words on the issues in emergency care, but I'm sure that the bulk of my *gestalt* (what Americans call the diagnostic 'hunch') has come from just engaging with so many humans, up close and personal. I'm equally sure that this initially mysterious intuition can be learned by anyone willing to spend many hours practising three core skills: courtesy, concentration and compassion.

Courtesy really means civility, politeness and consideration, and involves the suspension of self-interest. It means *actively* putting the patient at the top of one's immediate agenda and ignoring one's own needs as far as possible. Concentration incorporates attentiveness to and *awareness* of the patient, their appearance and everything that can be actively gleaned about them. Compassion is often misinterpreted as just a *feeling* of empathy, sympathy or kindness, but in medicine it must be combined with *action* as in the 'compassion equation': *compassion = empathy + action*. That really is my favourite definition of emergency healthcare.

The ability to practise courtesy, concentration and compassion reflects both moral and mental awareness. Consider this telling psychological study. In 1999, psychologists Christopher Chabris and Daniel Simons devised an experiment in which six people are videoed playing with basketballs. Three of the people are wearing white tops, three are wearing black tops, and as they move around in a circle throwing the balls at each other, a large gorilla walks from the right of the screen into the centre of the circle of players, thumps his chest and then exits, stage left.

When viewers were asked in advance to count the number of passes of the ball made by the players, it transpired that roughly half of them failed entirely to see the gorilla, who spent a full nine seconds on screen. It's an amusing example of a trick of the mind, but in psychological terms it reveals two things: we miss a lot of what goes on around us, and we have no idea that we are missing so much. Technically, this is called *inattentional blindness*, and curing it in the course of a doctor's training is where the real magic of medicine comes in, I believe. In a way, it involves the deepest possible interest in what is going on in a patient's mind, consciously and unconsciously, *and in the doctor's mind too*. It requires endless practice, but much of it can be described as common sense.

The primary, key, essential skill to be learned here is *empathy*. This begins as *genuinely caring* for someone and wanting to help them. It proceeds to *mirroring* their emotions, by discerning what is going on in the other's (the patient's) mind. This is helped by *blurring the boundaries* between the doctor and the patient, the key goal being to communicate to the other (the patient) that their innermost feelings are *recognised*. But it must be done with exquisite sensitivity, and the 'recognition' needs to be conveyed in a way that the patient can accept, without feeling judged, despised or ridiculed. Hence, it is crucial that the doctor understands the way that people (patients) reach decisions. This is because it is so often the consequences of flawed or illogical decisions that bring people to an emergency department. 'What were you *thinking?*' is arguably the worst question to put to a patient. Trust me.

I think that all doctors are 'privileged' in this context, so they must appreciate that the reason why patients make certain decisions comes down simply to their life story. I am very keen on this idea. On the one hand, I believe that doctors who have had their own little difficulties in life may have a bit more empathy. On the other hand, and this is fundamental, *difficulty makes people difficult*. This is the most important conclusion I've reached in my career as a would-be Samaritan, and it is one I quietly recalled whenever I felt worn out by the carry-on of some people I met during the course of a shift in the ED. I suppose, ironically, emotional trauma can in a sense be contagious.

Repeating this mantra about difficulty reminds me that the patient in front of me, who has turned up in the crammed emergency department drunk or full of heroin, Paracetamol or sleeping pills for the third time in a week, is there for a reason. And the reason is not 'for fun'. The explanation, if sought, is very often that their parents were addicted to alcohol, heroin, benzodiazepines or violence, and their childhood may have featured separation, starvation, physical, sexual or mental brutality every day of their young lives. The patient, who may be terribly scarred, literally or figuratively, has often spent their childhood studying a dysfunctional adult figure upon whom, like all offspring, they are biologically dependent.

That kind of 'home schooling' may lead to an imitation of their role model and their habits. Fr Peter McVerry, the indefatigable activist who's been battling homelessness and deprivation in Ireland since the 1970s, talks of serving a 'third generation' of Dublin heroin addicts, and the hereditary nature of the resulting misery. My experience in both the UK and Ireland offers ample proof of that. And I can confirm that the most difficult patients of all are the ones with the most hideous family histories. Like the elderly male who presents every second day to a different ED having pulled off yet another dressing on his leg that had taken a public health nurse an hour to apply, so he could tear through the healing ulcers with his fingernails. I'm describing a real case as anonymously as I can because many of these patients are utterly exasperating, and very, very hard to manage. The CDU sees many such cases of teenage girls who self-harm after being abused, and of course abused boys will abreact and get into trouble with the law and pitch up to the ED, often in the back of a police van having punched or head-butted walls. And even the heroin addicts who are perpetually robbing the ED staff lockers in many hospitals are doing it because they crave the oblivion which eases the ghastly memories they must otherwise carry around in their head. My point is that, if medics really want to *care* for the patient in front of them, they must suspend both disbelief and judgement for the duration, and work on getting into the shoes of the other. Even if there *are* a lot of shoes.

And while there are many simple ways in which doctors can empathise with their patients, there are always pitfalls. I always used to give my patients a firm handshake, as I'd been taught to do as a boy, until one day, I met a gentle middle-aged lady who'd presented with a sore leg. As always, I said, 'Hello, my name is Chris, I'm one of the doctors here. Can I offer you a seat and a glass of water?' I pulled over the chair, proffered a paper cup of cold water, as was my habit, and I shook her hand. At which point she screamed, 'Ouch, my hand!' She didn't quite shout, 'You brute!' at me, but I was quite taken aback and wondered if she was a little over-sensitive, even if the consultation was otherwise uneventful. Now, ten years on, I have my own damaged nerves and arthritis, so I understand better. The last time I met my friend, Paul Byrne, the congenial TV3 reporter, I got a taste of my own medicine when he shook my hand firmly and I let out an involuntary yelp of pain. Looking back, I realise that empathy must be about the conscious *and* the subconscious plus a good helping of *common sense*.

The ideal patient consultation puts the patient at their ease with an introduction, a chair, a well-judged handshake or, in COVID times, an elbow tap. Then preliminary information-gathering can begin. If they speak English, it is important to engage in a little banter to establish that they understand what you are saying and vice versa. If they don't, an interpreter is essential. The same may apply to a chaperone. And, of course, cultural mores must be observed. Eye contact is important in Western societies but is regarded as rude in others, such as some Hispanic, Asian, Middle Eastern and Native American cultures. The rules of engagement may reflect the global movement of people, but the fundamentals remain the same. Profound respect, courtesy and consideration are prerequisites of all patient-doctor contacts.

Patient comfort must be addressed before any longer conversation. Clearly, the critically sick or injured must be treated immediately, even if they are unconscious or incapable of communicating. Otherwise, once the patient is seated, the water is sipped and the chaperone or interpreter is in place, the doctor's task is to reduce their distress. Again, simple rules apply. By definition, being a patient is distressing because one feels at the mercy of the system, or the professional, often fearful or physically distressed. In a busy emergency department, there isn't much time for philosophising, so I cling to a phrase I first saw as a young doctor (and which does have ancient origins): *Happiness is the absence of pain.* That's it. Forget complex belief systems. Just make sure people are not in unnecessary distress and focus on the ancient notion that happiness is the absence of pain.

I find that the vast majority of patients are *measurably* happier if they are seen reasonably promptly (or given a rough idea when they will be seen), they meet a doctor who is clearly concerned and who first says, 'What I want to do first is to make you as happy as possible by sorting out your pain.' Not those exact words, but that should clearly be the intention. I have little time for questions that go, 'On a scale of one to ten, can you rate your distress?' In my view, such queries are as reliable as general election voting intention or sex surveys. What doctors (and nurses) need to do is to proactively *recognise* the patient's distress. Surprisingly, this is an area in which younger healthcare professionals often initially lack aptitude, because medical education is so focused on textbook learning and diagnostic algorithms, rather than on 'soft skills' like empathy. But they need to learn quickly, because the primary purpose of an emergency department is to *alleviate suffering*, and *what you don't see, you don't treat.*

Distress is as variable as patients, naturally, and there are some West Cork farmers, front-row forwards and jockeys who seem oblivious of the pain that an obviously broken ankle, shoulder or ribcage is supposed to cause. Conversely, other patients roar with distress without obvious cause and it only transpires later that they are 'hospital hoppers', frequenting every institution in a city in turn to get a shot of opioid for their chronic habit. Most senior emergency physicians realise that the sooner you relieve pain, the sooner your patient is able to help you make a diagnosis. And, in truth, 'hospital hoppers' are rare, so even if someone tricks you into giving a shot of morphine, it is unlikely to do any harm.

The key to a good standard consultation is to administer water, paracetamol, anti-inflammatory or opioid medication as needed once the level of distress is calculated. And ranging from a sprained ankle to period pain to an imminent brain bleed to a ruptured aorta, there is a scale of visible distress, from wincing to gasping to bouncing off the bed, which can be appreciated by a practised eye.

The assessment must not be one-dimensional, and increasing distress means that the wincing will be associated with pallor, crying, gasping, guarding of sore parts and changes in the vital signs, like rapid breathing or pulse. And the relief of the pain must be similarly rounded. I believe that giving someone a seat and some water, smiling reassuringly and being 'theatrically' kind can reduce the levels of distress by about 20 per cent. Anyone who has felt a parched throat while waiting for an interview or oral exam will appreciate the difference that a sip of cold water can make to the associated headache and stress. I have seen senior doctors flounder, pale-faced, on the brink of fainting at interview, until they were given a transformative glass of H_2O.

Effective pain relief, then, is about mind *and* body. It involves the *optics* of caring, a little pharmacology, and physiology. That is why just sipping, sitting, resting, turning the light out in a cubicle, splinting a sore limb, putting pressure on a bleeding wound, draining a tense collection of blood under a fingernail or a boil, elevating a swollen limb, slipping a pillow under a painful hip, or just holding a hand can all work wonders. Of course, *everyone* is under pressure in an emergency department, so I always urge staff to ask patients just one simple question, even if they're running off to someone even more distressed: 'Have you ever had a similar problem in this part of your anatomy before?' This one query can prevent frazzled professionals missing the clues to heart attacks, recurrent lung, kidney or bowel disease, slipped discs or sinister nerve disease, as well as remembering especially vulnerable anatomy following previous injury.

Again, the basis of medical magic is experience. For instance, it is said that, in general practice, over 80 per cent of diagnoses can be deduced from a medical history alone, and for those emergency department patients referred by their GPs, up to half of the letters will contain the correct diagnosis. And after the referral letter has been read, a systematic enquiry using simple checklists, with particular emphasis on legal or illegal medication or allergies, can usually identify most of the remaining clues.

Once the patient's issues have been prioritised in the initial conversation, the clinical examination can be undertaken. 'Clinical' is a word that seems to be most often heard on TV, when a striker pops a ball just past the goalkeeper's fingertips, but it actually derives from the French word *clinique*, which in turn is based on the Greek *klinike tekhne*, meaning bedside. And that's what it really means. It refers to the *location* of the patient, on a chair, couch or trolley, and it traditionally refers to the aspect of patient care that does not involve much of what we nowadays call technology, or kit.

Once a doctor has passed the 10,000-patient mark, they will often have a surprisingly good *gestalt* or 'gut feeling' in terms of patients' problems. Studies have suggested that a step-change also occurs at around the fifth year after graduation, which comes down to pattern recognition by the now-more-experienced medics. The science suggests that the brain innately processes findings that are similar to a known pattern, even when the findings are incomplete. It might be described as 'joining the dots'.

Regardless of rank, the doctor will hopefully have done some preparation for the typical menu of presentations to an emergency department. They will also have been inducted into the initial treatments of such conditions, and if they are someone who likes to avoid failure, they will have carefully studied a textbook of surface anatomy. This is because a busy clinician has to appreciate what is *under their thumb*, no matter where they place it on the outside of a patient's body. If they don't know, they shouldn't really treat patients. That sounds harsh, but almost every aspect of diagnosis and care depends on recognising the affected anatomy. Actually, one of my favourite teaching sessions is what I call Desert Island

Diagnostics. This is a simple challenge to trainees to come up with the likeliest anatomical diagnosis in every square inch of the body, using just their ears, eyes and hands. And strictly *no* magic wands!

The first real diagnostic test in terms of the doctor's touch is, of course, the *handshake* itself, which can reveal a great deal about a patient: from the strength and bulk of their muscles to the integrity and control of the nerves between brain and fingertips, to painful conditions like arthritis, infection or injury anywhere on their upper limb and neck. Experience suggests that it is possible to roughly gauge *longevity*, the presence of *malnutrition* and the general ability to *cooperate* (which reflects brain function, consciousness and culture) from the way a patient grips the doctor's hand. Using their fingers and thumb, the doctor can then work out precisely where the greatest tenderness or other abnormality is on the surface of the patient. This often identifies the relevant area of *inflammation* (meaning redness, heat, swelling and pain), *injury* (like a bruise, fracture or slipped intervertebral disc) or any other *interesting issue*. Mind you, what most patients don't really want to hear from their doctor is the word 'interesting', especially if it is followed by an intake of breath or repeated whistling through teeth. What we all much prefer is something obvious, simple and easily sorted.

Once the experienced clinician has identified the bit under their thumb that is sore, swollen or otherwise amiss, they should be able to name the adjacent anatomy, be it skin, skeletal or deeper still, and that will generally suggest the diagnosis. When multiple bits are affected, the doctor must reach for *pattern recognition* and what they recall from the textbooks. Most of the time, however, in an emergency department, a *working diagnosis* can be reached without the use of any technology, and the radiologists, laboratory scientists and other specialists are only involved when there is something serious or sinister suspected. Even then, most further tests are done ideally to *confirm* the clinical suspicion.

After that, most of the time all that remains is for the doctor to assist nature in the healing process, with initial painkillers, steroids or antibiotics, splintage or drainage, and rest. The best-kept secret in medicine is that most ailments and injuries resolve with time. As Voltaire, the great French sage, said, 'The art of medicine consists of amusing the patient while nature cures the disease'. I couldn't agree more. We know that with topical ice, heat, simple pain relief and rest, most sports injuries will settle within a few weeks. Even uncomplicated fractures are usually on the way to healing within six weeks or so, once protected from knocks or too much weight-bearing. Most tension headaches will evaporate with a little water, a laugh and a good sleep, while many surface infections, like pustules, will settle with simple occlusion (covering them with a band-aid) and perhaps a few days' antibiotics. And viral illnesses usually settle at home, as long as there aren't sinister signs, like difficulty in breathing, impaired consciousness, cold fingers and toes, or unbearable pain.

One of the great myths in first aid is that a sleeping patient must be roused regularly after a head injury to 'check if they are okay'. In fact, sleep is Mother Nature's way of sorting most minor ailments. I'd love to be able to think up some really simple rule of thumb to distinguish between what's really serious and what's not, but alas it comes back to experience. A good first-aider will know, as will most emergency department veterans. But the one thing I will say to everybody is that *no one knows a child better than their mother*. If she says her baby is not right, then *she's always right*. Until proven otherwise. And that particularly applies to nasty illnesses like meningitis, heart failure or diabetes. If a mum says, 'He's not been himself for the past two weeks,' I get much more alarmed than if he was 'grand' the night before.

If all of this sounds ridiculously time-consuming, it isn't, once you get the hang of it. I have rehearsed this approach to my patients for decades, and I've compressed the introduction, relief and initial assessment of most patients into just two or three minutes. If you set aside the time needed for an x-ray or occasional blood test in caring for most ED patients, and the time needed for dressings, bandaging, plastering or stitches, most of which should be done within about 90 minutes in a well-organised service, I think that a really effective emergency medical consultation could take as little as five minutes prior to diagnosis, treatment planning and delivery.

There is one other key ingredient in the ideal patient consultation: written information. We've known for decades that the vast majority of patients forget what the doctor said by the time they get back to their car, bicycle or bus. So I write down the key take-home message on a simple paper slip for them. 'Your problem is: a suspected microfracture of the scaphoid wrist bone. The plan is: return for review in this emergency department at 15.40 hrs on 10.03.2019', and so on. I reckon this adds two minutes to each consultation, but I'm sure it's done more than any other intervention in my long career to enhance patient satisfaction, and it greatly reduced the 'DNA' (did not attend) rate at my clinics. In financial terms, I believe it has saved my hospitals thousands of euro in a small number of claims which were rebutted once it was shown that the instructions on the information cards differed from what was subsequently alleged.

Frankly, if I were Minister for Health, this is the one cheap intervention I would introduce everywhere: a sort of print-out after every outpatient medical consultation, which can so easily prevent misunderstandings and breakdowns in communication. Those breakdowns can cost the health service a fortune, not to mention the distress to patients and doctors due to misunderstandings. And if I am honest, while I think that the advances in healthcare technology over the past 40 years have been truly awesome, I can still think of nothing more rewarding in the course of a patient's visit to an ED than transforming their face from fearful, tearful and pale, to cheerful, beaming and pink. I really do believe it's a kind of magic.

Shattered Dreams

One of the more disconcerting things I've noticed in recent years, as I gradually became an 'OEP', or older emergency physician, is that so many of the once-familiar faces in my speciality, people who I trained under or with, have disappeared. Of course, a few have died tragically prematurely, but the vast majority seem to have just shuffled off and, like old soldiers, faded away. The number of colleagues who have left the stage early is very considerable, and I'm pretty certain, given the stories circulating within our relatively small community, that a good proportion were driven by so-called 'burnout', or that spiritual exhaustion due to stressful work and shattered dreams.

Burnout is a term that is frequently bandied about, but it demands serious examination. The first thing to understand is that the World Health Organisation (WHO) redefined it in 2019 as an *occupational health syndrome*, resulting from chronic workplace stress that has not been successfully managed. The word *syndrome* refers to a combination of key features, such as physical, emotional and spiritual exhaustion accompanied by disabling cynicism and despondency. Put at its simplest, sufferers feel 'stuck, exhausted and hopeless'.

The longer burnout is left unmanaged, the more damaging it becomes to the person's performance, physical and mental well-being and, perhaps most significantly, to their *relationships* at work and home. What I have found most troubling is the way burnout has moved like a silent epidemic through the medical profession for the past twenty years, a period that coincides with the disintegration of my own once-promising career. The second most important thing to understand is that burnout is not another name for depression or 'endogenous melancholia', or whatever. As the late, lamented Professor Anthony Clare once explained to me, occupational stress among doctors poses a very real threat because, while antidepressant medication is a potential remedy for the *secondary* symptoms of burnout like anguish and despair, it is not a *cure* for the underlying disease. What he hinted at, and what I have learned as I've studied the condition, is that it seems to be *cured* only by leaving the workplace that is causing it. That may sound like an unreasonable, if not histrionic, assertion, and I actually resisted it for years, but the statistics are sobering. In the past few years, systematic studies in the USA, UK, Australasia and Ireland (where healthcare systems are so similar that medics move freely between them) have found that between a third and a half of doctors are experiencing serious levels of burnout. Some surveys have suggested even higher proportions, but I think the conservative figures I've indicated are reasonably reliable.

The Medical Protection Society is the leading medical indemnity (or professional insurance) provider for doctors in

Ireland and when it comes to significance among the medical profession, it is probably on a par with the Medical Council or medical Royal Colleges. The MPS surveyed its members in Ireland in 2019 and found that almost half these doctors had considered leaving the profession because of unhappiness, most felt unsupported in their workplace, over 40 per cent were dissatisfied with their work-life balance and worn out at the start of their working day, and 30 per cent often felt unable to get away from the shopfloor for a tea or a pee. In short, there were a lot of unhappy doctors. And it's much the same across the Irish Sea, where 'physician morale is at an all-time low', according to a contributor to the *Lancet* in 2020.

But surveys are one thing and facts are different. Which is why, when it comes to voters or doctors, I always ask: so what did they *do* in the end? And what doctors are doing should come as a shock to those who run – or use – the public health service in Ireland, the UK, or even New Zealand, which is so popular with younger doctors in the Northern Hemisphere but where two-thirds of female doctors are now said to be suffering from burnout. What they are doing is jumping ship.

Commentators in Ireland can sometimes get a bit parochial about the 'churn' in medical employment here, but the fact is that the underlying drivers of medical attrition are much the same everywhere in the English-speaking world. In the UK, the number of so-called F2 (second postgraduate year) doctors applying to continue with their specialist training in the NHS has fallen from over 70 per cent in 2011 to about 38 per cent in 2018, while the number of doctors taking career breaks from the NHS has risen to nearly 15 per cent, or about one in seven. These figures are staggering once you realise that the NHS is *already* short of about 10,000 doctors. And they are even more worrying if you consider that the doctors most at risk of burnout and its complications are female intensive care specialists or GPs in their late 40s onwards. The gendered part, of course, may be the added domestic duties that often fall to women. At the moment, over 70 per cent of GP trainees in Ireland are female, while about a third of anaesthetists (the speciality that produces sub-specialist intensivists) are female. And talking of being parochial, I don't just worry about the implications of this for patients and healthcare staff 'out there', I fret as the father of a dynamic and highly dedicated medical daughter with an interest in critical care.

The reality, then, is that both the Irish health service and the NHS are in the grip of a longstanding workforce crisis.

We already know that there are hundreds of vacant hospital consultant posts in the Republic of Ireland, and every year a considerable proportion of our new medical graduates leave the country to work abroad. In 2021, the exodus is predicted to increase to unprecedented levels, and the IMO has suggested that as many as 600 young doctors will leave Ireland during 2021 due to a lack of Intern (first year) posts here, or because the working conditions are regarded as intolerable. Not surprisingly, graduates prefer in the main to work Down Under, where the pressure, prospects and pay are all much more agreeable, for now.

Meanwhile, in the UK, there are fewer GPs than ever per head of population since the 1960s, countless nurse vacancies, and 10 per cent of specialist medical and over 30 per cent of psychiatry training posts are unfilled. The trends are similar in Ireland, and the result is a vicious cycle of low morale and burnout, much of it felt in the emergency department, where we've had difficulty recruiting younger doctors for decades. The result for those left working in an under-resourced service is very tough working conditions, which can lead, of course, to distress, disillusionment and, in time, burnout.

The causes of burnout are many and varied. The best-known authority on the subject is Christina Maslach, Professor Emerita of Psychology at the University of California at Berkeley, and author of the *Maslach Burnout Inventory*. She usefully identified six 'domains', or factors, that may contribute to the development of burnout: *workload* (too much), *control over work* (too little), *reward for work* (money alone is not enough), *sense of community* (not being isolated), *fairness* (and unfair treatment) and *values* (altruism can be crushed by capitalism and socialism).

Another type of cause is political, like the healthcare 'reforms' in the UK in the late 1980s by then-Health Secretary Ken Clarke. His 'back of a cigarette packet' plan to introduce the Thatcherite internal market to the NHS was soon followed by the *Patients' Charter*, which set out patients' rights and was said to have led to an increasing number of attacks on NHS staff. But everywhere in the English-speaking medical firmament, doctors moaned about the intrusion of capitalism, consumerism and complaint culture into healthcare.

This takes us back to the original problem and what to do about it. The reason why burnout among doctors matters is because *the burnt-out doctor doesn't care as much as he or she once dreamed of caring*. Unhappy doctors and nurses cannot provide the amount or quality of concern that their patients may need. I would be wary of attending a doctor who was suffering from severe occupational stress, because he or she is more likely to make mistakes of judgement, to pose a greater therapeutic risk and to have less empathy. Not to put too fine a point on it, burnout in healthcare professionals is a prescription for very unsatisfactory patient consultations.

I personally think that capitalism and consumerism play a large part. In the *British Medical Journal* of 16 November 1996, Noman Browse, Past President of the Royal College of Surgeons of England, and Stephen Eisenstein, a busy orthopaedic surgeon, both wrote opinion pieces about the rapid decline in medics' morale brought about by the cultivation of unreasonable *expectations* of doctors combined with a loss of independence and control over their workload. And in the Southern Hemisphere, physicians worried about the splintering of the profession by ultra-specialisation and competing professional agendas, combined with a new culture of individualism, full of mistrust of institutions and professionals in general. And, for decades now, American analysts have been complaining about the ruinous cost of healthcare in the USA, which recent writers say is 'literally killing people' in its pursuit of profit. Already, by December 2000, healthcare managers everywhere were talking of a 'hyperturbulent' healthcare environment, with an 'unsettling organizational climate' due to a proliferation of rival stakeholders.

Many of these political, commercial, regulatory and managerial reforms were imported willy-nilly into Ireland over the past 30 years. I have often thought that Irish policymakers always seemed to be keen to introduce a model of management from overseas, just when that model had been seen to fail in the original setting. One egregious example of this was then Minister for Health James Reilly's idea that we should copy 'the Dutch model' of healthcare. He told the *Irish Times* in

March 2010 that he had seen it for himself and had actually 'stood in the AE department with no trolleys'. But I too have stood in amazement in a Dutch emergency department and wondered why it was so quiet, until I realised that the way the health system there works is totally different from that in Ireland. I have worked in and visited the Netherlands often enough to understand that they are a very different people from the Irish. Not only are they taller, blonder and better at football, they spend more on healthcare, they have mandatory private health insurance to cover primary and secondary care, and they had 24-hour primary care clinics and telemedicine long before the current pandemic, resulting in a very different approach to 'emergencies'. Even so, by 2012 there were growing complaints about overcrowding in Dutch EDs and anxiety about the level of training of doctors within them.

The new NHS hospital consultants' contract in the UK in 2003 was another classic example of premature imitation in Ireland. The imposition of the contract, which had been vigorously resisted by consultants, was found a few years later by the Public Accounts Committee in Westminster to have resulted in a collapse in morale, productivity and creativity among NHS consultants, who were now subjected to rigid micromanagement. And the independent *King's Fund*, in the UK, which monitors such matters, published a report in 2006 which said about the very controversial contract: 'the cost of implementation has been greater than anticipated or budgeted for … because the funding formula was based on flawed financial and workload assumptions'. It had detrimentally affected consultants' 'professionalism' (i.e. autonomy, choice and relatedness) and there was 'little sign as yet that the patient care benefits envisaged are being realised'.

The political response on this side of the Irish Sea, five years later, was *not to learn* about the lamentable impact of the 2003 NHS deal, but to foist a remarkably similar new contract on consultants here. It was so focused on straitjacketing consultants, by reducing their private practice and micromanaging their workload, that it is arguably the primary cause of the 700-plus vacancies in the country today. Unfortunately, such initiatives are seldom occasions for transparent and polite debate, and often seem to involve the art of war rather than conciliatory diplomacy. One of the particularly disheartening pieces of propaganda that was put out, at the time of the 2008 negotiations between doctors and the government, was that the contract was only trying to get consultants to work 'out-of-hours', which as anyone who works in a hospital will know is a deeply offensive absurdity. For decades, all over this country, there have been consultants hard at work in hospitals every day and night of the year. Mostly this is because they must sort out emergencies, or their operations or procedures lists have overrun. But one key reason why there aren't more consultants working late at night and over the weekend in our hospitals is that many institutions simply cannot afford the operating theatres, imaging facilities or support staff needed to enable consultants to undertake the kind of specialist work they do. In practice, for decades, consultants have had to beg for such resources, occasionally going to the press to make their case or, worst of all, waiting for a coroner's or a lawyer's description of the scandalous deficits in facilities or imaging available outside normal working hours in a hospital to hit the papers.

It would be nice if those who are introducing complicated or wide-ranging initiatives into the system took the time to learn from history, and *to see what has or hasn't worked elsewhere*. More importantly, they might look at the sheer complexity and number of conflicting and contradictory demands on health service staff at all levels, and at least think twice about the latest imported idea.

So, have any of the ideas worked to help alleviate the problem of burnout? Many 'fixes' have been prescribed, and I have personally benefitted from a few, like the free massage sessions for staff at the Royal Liverpool University Hospital. But I really wish that those who, for instance, prescribe 'mindfulness' to enhance staff resilience understand that *it is the workplace that is making doctors and nurses sick*, not the want of moral fibre implied by 'mind games'. And the workplace is what needs fixing.

Incidentally, I think that team nights out, free makeovers, discounts in local salons, classes in philosophy or gardening, walking the Comeraghs, and summer parties are all *great* ways of improving staff morale. But they should be the icing on the cake. People need to appreciate that the staff in EDs around these islands are often individuals who are exceptionally hardworking, humane, and even heroic. What they rarely are is wimpish, neurotic or feeble. If anything, ED doctors and nurses are unusually dedicated, values-driven and *more* resilient than staff in more peaceful parts of the health system.

The Maslach Burnout Inventory (a tick-box exercise) is one way of diagnosing burnout, but there are simpler ways. In 2015, my colleague, Gerard White, an Advanced Nurse Practitioner at CUH, completed his PhD on the question of 'moral distress', which is what results when a healthcare professional *knows* what is the right thing to do but is *prevented* from doing it by institutional constraints. In practice, Ger found that ED staff everywhere *dream* of doing the right thing, and they train to do it, often brilliantly, but they end up unable to deliver such care due to a lack of resources. So they find themselves, like hamsters on a wheel, working ever harder to achieve less and less, and eventually realise they are actually rationing care on behalf of their institution. This recognition often represents the end-stage of 'compromised care', with exhausted staff avoiding eye contact with patients waiting in corridors for hours and trying not to burst into tears at the cacophony of pleas for their attention. The net result is that, having finally realised that their dedication and *dreams* have all come to naught, the staff quit the ED, taking with them years of training, experience and wisdom.

A third way of looking at burnout is to examine what makes certain types of work appealing to people. In medicine, as in other professions, the three drivers of motivation were once said to be *autonomy, complexity* and *meaning.* These were the basic reasons I chose a career in emergency medicine. Once fully trained, it meant that I was an *independent* actor, the work was *interesting,* and it provided me with a real sense of *doing the right thing,* at least within the value system that I clung to (a rather old-fashioned combination of social justice, fairness and decency). And those metrics really worked for me until I was about 40, I reckon. More recently, American commentators on burnout have refined the drivers of motivation as *autonomy, competence* and *relatedness.* Autonomy is having independence and choice in what you decide. Competence is a deep fund of medical skill, experience and *gestalt,* which enable you to make a clinical judgement. Relatedness is a sense of belonging to a community, as in the ED community. But they have added a further twist to their definition. They divided motivation into *intrinsic* and *extrinsic*. The former is about doing something because it is deeply interesting and personally meaningful, while the latter is about external rewards, like money.

In a profoundly important study, in 2005, Gagni and Deci discovered that 'intrinsic motivation is not only much more important to occupational satisfaction, but too much emphasis on external motivation can paradoxically undermine intrinsic motivation'.

In other words, too much focus on money or filling in financial claim forms can be demotivating. Because *meaning* really is more important than money. The researchers were studying the American healthcare system, of course, which is largely driven by the profit motive and rigid insurer-determined treatment algorithms. Many doctors there spend hours filling out electronic healthcare records so that 'performance indicators' can be recorded. The result is that autonomy, judgement, meaning and a sense of belonging are all shrivelling. And in that context, burnout is surging.

So what can be done, on a practical level? Well, first, we need to acknowledge that burnout is a huge and growing problem in our healthcare system, and we need to agree that it must be addressed with sensitivity and urgency. I think that those who are in a position to help ED staff need to do something that may make them uncomfortable. They need to *visit* the staff's workplace regularly, to study the workflow (or lack thereof), the staffing levels and the ergonomics. They need to ask themselves: are the instruments, drugs and technology needed to treat patients adequate and easily accessible? Is the place filthy, overcrowded and frightening? And then, be they politician, manager, specialist colleague or policy-maker, they need to be *proactively* helpful.

As always, history offers parallels and potential solutions. In 1889, Sir William Osler, the celebrated Canadian physician, gave a valedictory address to the latest medical graduates of the University of Pennsylvania. He described the most important quality of any physician as *imperturbability*, by which he meant 'coolness and presence of mind under all circumstances … and clearness of judgment in moments of grave peril'. Its opposite, Osler said, was 'indecision and worry' or an appearance of being 'flustered and flurried in ordinary emergencies', which 'loses rapidly the confidence of patients'. This external imperturbability needed to be matched by an *inner mental placidity*, which he called 'a calm equanimity'. One difficulty with this prescription was prompted by Osler himself in another context when he suggested that doctors over the age of 60 (like me!) were essentially past their best-by date. But I really agree with Sir William about the 'optimal' medical mindset. I think emergency physicians tend to reach peak performance before their mid-40s and, given that the challenge of difficult ED working conditions is unlikely to become easier any time soon, I think that some fresh thinking is required. Again, I borrow from the past. If we were to study the last quarter-century of ED staffing in the islands, I think it is likely we could work out the current average length of stay of staff nurses and younger doctors. I believe we could then find the *typical* and the *ideal* tenure of medical and nursing staff at the frontline.

And then, and this is my main solution to burnout among ED staff, we could implement a 'Tour of Duty' concept, or *limited tenure*. I constantly remind people that emergency medicine is the offspring of military medicine and missionary medicine and that, crucially, neither of these careers tends to be for the whole of a working life. In fact, most military or missionary tours of duty are *finite*. This is because it is recognised that military and missionary frontline staff need regular R&R time, as well as relatively early retirement. Such early retirement already tends to happen in our military and police forces, and even in the ranks of psychiatry, because the innate stress and corrosion associated with such work is *explicitly* recognised in contracts. And already, in the UK and elsewhere, there has been considerable debate about taking older emergency physicians off the on-call roster after the age of, say, 55 years. This should have happened years ago, in my view.

But I believe (and hope) that the future of emergency nursing and emergency medicine means that a career in the healthcare frontline will be mostly for young people (including perhaps a twelve-month stint for every graduate) and will typically last about ten to fifteen years, with a tapering-off for older physicians and nurses and a dialling down of their workload intensity, as both flesh and spirit become weaker. Paradoxically, such a reduction in their burden could actually allow older staff to work for longer, and perhaps to pursue their secondary dreams. The alternative, continuing as we are, is simply the definition of madness, and means that we continue endlessly to squander the experience and energies of young and old. It will perpetuate avoidable misery for all within the EDs, as well as a shocking waste of time, energy and money constantly trying to recruit new staff or temporarily replace sick staff.

I like to think that the very opposite of burnout is Osler's *equanimity*. And I really hope that I exhibited such equanimity in the case of 'ordinary emergencies', like cot deaths, cardiac arrest or gunshot wounds to the chest. But the very opposite applied to my response to the everyday working conditions. What I found endlessly *perturbing* throughout my entire career was the suffocating congestion in most EDs and the resulting corrosion of nurses' and doctors' ambitions and hopes. In this respect, I continue to resist *imperturbability* when it comes to overcrowded EDs, which can look dangerously like indifference. So I urge politicians and policymakers to try to understand the many non-medical problems in EDs and work ceaselessly to address them so that the staff and patients within can have at least an adequate and comfortable experience. Even if they have no great personal enthusiasm in tackling the issues, they might at least recall that the performance of an ED hugely affects the confidence of the local population in their health service. And at every election time, I would recommend that *every voter should ask their local TD when they were last in the local ED*.

The takeaway message about burnout and its well-known and often obvious causes is that ED doctors' and nurses' primary function is to *care*. They cannot do this *and* mind dozens of patients waiting for a bed, *and* all the other stuff that is so often delegated to them. Like filling more and more forms, ordering stock, begging for beds or assistance from a specialist colleague, cleaning the floor again, finding chairs upstairs, answering phones, restraining the violent patient at the ambulance door, hunting down some sandwiches and tea for the elderly diabetic who's been in Cubicle 3 since yesterday, chasing the teenage self-harmer that no one will admit … and on and on and on. Sure, changes that 'tweak' the workspace may help for a time. But when the staff are overwhelmed, there are ultimately two choices: they can obtain at least some of the assistance or resources that they need, including a clear impression that they are *respected*; or they can be *ignored* until they leave.

And when I say all of this – and when I go on so much about burnout – believe me, it's because it's *personal* and serious, and I really do know what I am talking about.

The Elephant in the Room

From the very start, I will now admit, I found my job straddling three hospitals in Cork as impossible as I'd been warned it would be. And it got worse. It was incredibly draining, having to rotate constantly between three different emergency departments, but my natural enthusiasm – and my reluctance to say 'no' – meant my working days became relentlessly ever-more crowded.

As a medical educationalist at CUH, I was dealing with Royal College and Medical Council inspections, running the Intern Teaching Programme every Tuesday, running the CUH Grand Rounds every Wednesday, and planning and hosting the Final MB Clinical Skills Course each summer for the 100-odd medical graduates of UCC. And, by way of extracurricular work, I was engaged in the RCSI trauma project, which was hugely time-consuming, as was the Club Cork programme I'd helped to set up. I had also launched the Cork Emergency Medicine Forum, a quarterly gathering in the elegant Maryborough Hotel which provided an enjoyable opportunity for staff from all around Munster to meet and exchange ideas, but which again entailed a lot of preparation. As if all that wasn't enough, I was busy with lecture commitments hither and yon.

It was clearly an excessive workload, especially as I was pretty worn out from the daily hand-to-hand combat in the EDs and their offices. And, of course, the 'politics' of healthcare, where it is not the issues or debateable facts but egos that matter. It was obvious by then that my great mistake had been to take a job in three rival hospitals. But having accepted my fate, my second error was to try to carve out an autonomous identity within my contractual straitjacket. Sadly, I had realised from the outset that I would never again win the affection of an entire emergency department crew, given that I could seldom linger in any of my three departments. Already, by early 2000, I had resigned myself to a life of endless commuting between hospitals. However, I still felt the same impulse that had driven me in Liverpool to evangelise, or to make people aware of the difficulties faced in the country's overcrowded emergency departments, particularly in relation to injury care, poisoning and paediatrics, my areas of interest. So I blithely pursued opportunities or accepted invitations to speak, write or lecture about these topics when they arose, as they did periodically.

In the end, it was somebody else – who perhaps should have said 'no' years previously – who saved the day and salvaged my career in Cork. More than anyone else, my long-suffering wife, Victoria (as Vicky was now called affectionately by her family), had put up with the vagaries of her husband's crazy career in emergency medicine, his obsessions, compulsions and intense insecurity. But one of the many advantages she possessed was real experience of a hectic A&E department, and the effect working in one can have on staff. She was also familiar with my anxieties and capacity to catastrophise. So, despite her own struggles as a Scottish immigrant, she concluded that the situation was not actually catastrophic. It was merely calamitous.

Brilliantly, as it turned out, she realised that there was only one thing that the Lukes *could* control in this new 'hyperturbulent' stage of their lives, and that was where we lived. It turned out to be an epiphany. One day in spring 2000, as she wandered home after leaving the girls into their new school, Eglantine, in Ballinlough, she stopped to study the houses for sale in the window of Marian Rose Auctioneers on the Douglas Road. There, that morning, and for weeks after, she noticed an advert for a house on the Castlemary Estate in East Cork, on the Whitegate road near Cloyne. The house was set in woodland in an old Anglo-Irish demesne, whose 'Big House' was one of many burned down in the strife of the 1920s, but it was now an area of exceptional tranquillity, at the tip of one of Cork Harbour's inlets, Saleen Creek.

It didn't take Victoria long to drive out to see it with one of her new girlfriends, and to take an executive decision that the extraordinary Park House, once home to the legendary entomologist Cynthia Longfield, or 'Madam Dragonfly', was precisely the sanctuary her faltering spouse needed, as well as our three 'square-eyed' girls. Another unexpected challenge we'd found on our return to a modern Irish housing estate in Cork was the numerous cable television channels available, in contrast with the handful in Liverpool. And both she and I had been aghast at the way the girls would close the curtains in our sitting room and spend entire days gawking at American TV, before emerging, blinking, into the light, only after their father got home. And I loudly lamented the dumbing-down of the children as they abandoned their previous love of reading for *Rugrats* and other 'rubbish', as I grumpily (and unreasonably) put it.

So when, in mid-summer 2000, my wife suddenly proposed 'moving to the countryside', it may well have been one of her usual *faits accomplis,* but I genuinely thought it sounded like a great idea. Especially when she explained that it was so remote, there would be *no* TV. In fact, such was our enthusiasm to make another fresh start that we ended up leaving our rented city house months earlier than planned and moving lock-stock to Park House.

There we spent a blissful and truly transformational eighteen months hiding in the native woodland of Castlemary as tenants, but feeling like guests, of the warm and generous owners, Des and Brid Hurley who, with their two boys, became great friends. In the evenings, after work, instead of negotiating the 'roundabout from hell', as I called the Kinsale Road junction, I would drive on east, past great fields of wheat and barley on my left and the green grandeur of Fota Island and the harbour on the right. In just twenty minutes or so, already breathing more easily, I would be bumping over the cattle grid at the Saleen gate and driving along the winding path through the woods. And 30 seconds later, the car would be crunching over the gravel outside the handsome Park House, with its terraces of exotic trees and shrubs planted by Madam Dragonfly herself. Best of all, in the final 50 yards of the drive, I usually glimpsed a rabbit in the long grass above the house, followed by a Luke girl or two leaping around happily, outside.

After fifteen years of urban living in Edinburgh and Liverpool, that period in East Cork felt like a vivid rural idyll.

The beginnings of burnout had been rumbling away in the background, ignored by me, but the relocation undoubtedly did more for my flagging spirits than any sun holiday or course in mindfulness could have done. A gentle jog along Saleen Creek on a summer's evening, listening to 'Navan Man' or John Creedon, provided the perfect antidote to a day navigating the chaos of an ED, and its attendant challenges. We also managed to attract a steady flow of visitors from Edinburgh, Liverpool, Dublin and Cork and it was a joy to see how many of them fell in love with our delightful hideaway and nearby gems, like Murph's Tavern in East Ferry, the pier in Aghada, and frankly everywhere between St Colman's Cathedral in Cloyne and Ballycotton. Best of all, the whole Luke family blossomed, especially my wife, who was pregnant with our fourth child, and first boy, a little Irishman with a 'sort of Scottish' name, Harrison.

Thanks to my wife's foresight and practicality, I was able to keep going and enjoy life with the family. But, acknowledged or not, the unrelenting nature of my work was taking its toll. I suppose we often mistake perseverance for stubbornness, and vice versa. Certainly, that was how I saw my tenaciousness at the time. But, as with madness and bright ideas, the dividing line can be treacherously blurred. I found this out very painfully in April 2001, in one of those life lessons that are never forgotten. Two decades on, I can still vividly relive the slow-motion car crash that was my lecture to the Surgical Section of the Royal Academy of Medicine, in Limerick, on Saturday, 21 April 2001.

I'd been slotted in at the start of the morning session, to give a talk on multiple trauma in Ireland, the deficiencies in its management and some of the remedies required for an effective national response. In truth, I'd planned to offer a sneak preview of the RCSI's *Clinical Guidelines*, then in preparation. Unfortunately, despite taking the Friday afternoon off to prepare for my talk in tranquil East Cork, I had fallen behind as a result of too many commitments at work and at home (where an infant boy was regularly disrupting his parents' sleep). In ominous military parlance, I had 'failed to prepare' and by the time I got to the hotel in Castletroy, I still had hours of work to do assembling a dual-slide presentation involving a ludicrous amount of images. The result was another entirely sleepless night, and it was only at about 7.30 a.m. on the Saturday that I was finalising the slide sequence.

Normally, I get into a venue early to make sure I'm acquainted with the layout, the projector and the podium, and I always run through the presentation, particularly one as complicated as my trauma talk that day. On this occasion, however, despite getting to the conference centre early, there was no one to let me in, and the technician arrived just moments before the kick-off was due. Even as he began to assist me, the audience of surgeons was already filling the auditorium, cheerfully chatting after their enjoyable late Friday night, and my anxiety was spiralling. I was used to feeling nervous and sweaty-palmed before starting a lecture, and usually a few deep breaths did the trick so by the second or third slide, I'd be into my stride. But, here, the projector still hadn't even been switched on by the time most of the seats were filled, and I think that appreciating that simple reality provoked that rare phenomenon, a total system failure. I was now exhausted, completely unsure of my slides, unacquainted with the auditorium, and the AV system was a nightmare. And then, in the crowd, I spotted some familiar faces, like

Niall O'Higgins and Gordon Watson, kindly elder statesmen of Irish surgery. But there were other, less sympathetic personalities I suddenly recalled from youthful encounters, and there was one particular face from Cork, the sight of which, alas, seemed to trigger a full-blown panic attack.

Most of us have probably read about stage fright. I certainly had, and I knew most of the tips for avoiding it, but on this occasion my inability to prepare was immaterial. I stood up as I was introduced and, looking out at all the expectant faces, I think I got to the third or fourth word of my preamble, when a white mist enveloped me. My voice dried up. Palpitations, breathlessness and a blinding headache overcame me and, with a squawked, 'I'm sorry, I don't feel …', I rushed off the stage, marched up the steps bisecting the audience, and out through the door of the conference centre. And I sat, hyperventilating and shaking my head in disbelief, on a bench outside.

I was vaguely aware of activity and bustle behind me, and a very solicitous Niall O'Higgins came out to see if I was alright, as did Arnie Hill, the up-and-coming academic surgeon who'd organised the event. But the rest of that day remains shrouded in a miserable haze. Eventually, my slides were retrieved and returned to me and the meeting continued. I made my way back to my hotel room, packed up and drove home, gasping and grief-stricken for my career as a lecturer, and my erstwhile hard-won confidence. Arriving home in Park House, I got straight into bed and had the deep, deep sleep I should have had the night before.

As ever, it was my wife and friends who kept me going that year. I recovered slowly from the calamitous maiden speech to the community of surgeons in Limerick, but despite a warm and heartfelt letter from Arnie Hill a few days later, and the unwavering support of Gordon Watson and Niall O'Higgins, the effects of that 'collapse of stout party' episode stayed with me for a very long time. The RCSI's *Clinical Guidelines on Initial Management of the Severely Injured Patient* was published a couple of years later, with a suitable fanfare in the College in Dublin, and I presented them at the CUH Grand Rounds, but I didn't feel able to trouble the surgical circuit again for a long time. Worst of all, I felt afterwards that the momentum generated in compiling the *Guidelines*, with their overview of – and prescription for – injury care in Ireland, was lost. Sadly, I still believe that they offered a substantial and useful contribution to the debate, and I like to think they made some difference. Mind you, given that the audit and the trauma centres prescribed in the RCSI *Guidelines* of 2003 are still 'imminent' in 2021, I no longer blame myself entirely, or my failure to prepare in 2001. Like any major crash experience, the angst induced by the events in Limerick coloured my professional and domestic life for years afterwards. I continued to adapt as best I could, relying as always on my eternally optimistic wife, and on the affection of friends old and new. But I found myself struggling intermittently for years, and eventually I sought occupational health support in 2007 for what I thought was 'self-evident' burnout, with the classical features of mental exhaustion, cynicism and crankiness due to relentless workplace stress.

Burnout is an extraordinarily interesting and important topic, unless you have it. Then, nothing seems very important or interesting. And when people ask you if you're alright, you say, 'Yeah, yeah. I'm just tired'. Or if they say, 'Chris, do you not think you need help?', you say, 'Maybe. I just need a break, really'. But you don't have the break, until serious damage is done, especially to relationships. In many ways, my career was a predictable casualty of severe 'spiritual anaemia', as I describe my own burnout. In other words, like an increasingly anaemic and iron-deficient patient, I was tired all the time, and unable to think.

My prospects had been quite decent, too, at least when I was in my thirties (and, in hindsight, at my peak). But in the years which followed that sudden crippling panic attack, the arc of my job was on a precipitously and painfully downward slope. I think I know where I went wrong, of course. First, choosing a crazy career at the healthcare frontline. Secondly, leaving a major NHS teaching hospital, where I was well placed for professional progress, to take up an absurd job straddling three institutions in a city that was unfamiliar to me. Thirdly, allowing myself to become isolated, politically and professionally. And, finally, sticking to my guns, to the deeply bitter end.

This meant that I started to squabble with colleagues over the direction of travel of our speciality in the city, over the relative staffing, resourcing and busyness of the three EDs, and over the sharing of the workload. In practice, it meant that I tended to 'firmly defend' the interests of the smaller departments against the dominance of the biggest teaching hospital and, inevitably, I began to fall out with some of the people at CUH who wanted 'more' of me there. And I began to fall out with some of the people at the Mercy who wanted 'more' of me there. In truth, I was getting very resentful of being pulled in different directions. And as I used to say jokingly to GPs, in those days when I gave them lectures, 'My gripe is bigger than your gripe'. So *everyone* felt hard done by, really.

I can't be certain, but I think that the fact that I was not coping must have been clear to my colleagues in the first six or seven years in Cork. Sadly, this was becoming manifest mostly in the squabbling I mentioned but, eventually, essential changes arrived incrementally, and I was 'permitted' to give up working at the South Infirmary in 2003. I also quit the medical education work in CUH in 2007, when I found I was unable to get the extra time or help I thought I needed to do it. Ironically, once I'd quit, the work of minding the Interns, running the Final MB Clinical Skills Course and chairing the Grand Rounds was handed to a number of other people. Happily, though, all of these activities were well bedded down, and they thrived 'under new management'.

I still struggled as the job of straddling two emergency departments, at the Mercy and CUH, continued to be difficult. Irony was heaped on irony when, in 2006, I had to say no to an invitation to become a 'Mercy only' consultant in the same year as a piece in the *Irish Medical Times* reported that the Accident and Emergency Task Force proposed to abolish the sort of 'shared post' between emergency departments that I had signed up to in 1999. The basic reason was that I wanted to minimise the risk of complete isolation away from the main hub of emergency medicine in CUH. A secondary reason was that I was sceptical that the Mercy management would invest the resources I'd pleaded for in their ED, and I suspected I would end up being on-call there 365 days a year.

Unfortunately, downsizing my commitments in terms of the number of EDs and 'extracurricular' educational work was still not enough to allow me to contend with the routine requirements of my two remaining EDs. Other stuff had to go, too. Small projects, like intriguing case reports, surveys of attitudes or performance, or studying the impact of certain interventions (medical audit), for instance, even if they are the bread-and-butter of medical education, markers of serious ambition and the prerequisites of an academic career. More than that, collaborating with trainees who sometimes undertake such work with real gusto is one of the great pleasures of a life in medicine. In my head, I think of it as combining the *rigour* of science with the *honest toil* of horticulture, and if it comes to fruition with a practice-changing paper, poster or presentation, it is hugely uplifting.

And so it was with a heavy heart that I eased myself away from anything more than the minimum of such activity after my first five years in Cork, but I just found it impossible to keep up with the staffing, training and political challenges of two emergency departments, as well as the clinical work. There were just too many patients to see, recruitment interviews to conduct, and committee meetings I couldn't miss (like the ones planning the new ED at the Mercy, or telling staff about the various major 'reforms' coming down the tracks from Dublin, London or New York).

While the changes did help, they were probably a sticking plaster for a problem that ran much deeper. By 2007, I'd downsized my duties as much as I could (without becoming a sort of isolated Robinson Crusoe in the Mercy Emergency Department), but I wasn't cured. It was clear that I needed to try a more professional approach to my issues. As my schoolfriend and lifelong *consigliere* David O'Donohoe is wont to say, 'Even Chris's issues have issues'. He and I had been at school since the 1960s, and he said that I was the only boy he'd ever known whose *surname* had suddenly changed, apparently after I discovered the letter from my father in 1970.

Before that there had been considerable uncertainty about my surname in my school, and in Oaktree Road, and I had used both my mother and father's surname interchangeably. And, looking back, it seems clear that I had begun to go off the rails, inside and outside school, after that time. So I'd long known that David was right about my 'issues', which may well have started with that identity crisis in 1970, and I'd often *contemplated* counselling or psychiatric therapy. But, like many middle-aged men carrying a great deal of baggage, I had always been 'too busy'.

Anyway, in the end, I was referred by Occupational Health for counselling, and I was given some antidepressant medication, which I tried for a while, pretty unsuccessfully. Indeed, my poor wife remembers one international conference we were at, in Sorrento, not long after I'd started the medication, and she says I was 'off my chump', as the Scots like to describe significant mental derangement. In fact, she was mortified because I behaved so 'oddly' when we'd bumped into old friends there from Edinburgh. Happily or unhappily, I can't remember this, but I gave up the medication PDQ, and returned to my status quo ante.

Regardless of the dodgy drugs, I readily agreed to see Professor Anthony Clare, the celebrated psychiatrist whose BBC Radio 4 programme, *In The Psychiatrist's Chair*, had been a favourite of mine during my time in the UK. I confess I'd had mixed views of psychiatry since my medical student days, when I had spent time studying the subject on an attachment at St John of God's Hospital and been struck by the then-limited range of demonstrably effective treatments for serious mental illness. Unfortunately, my view had also been shaped by the radical celebrity psychiatrists – or anti-psychiatrists – of the 1970s. These included RD Laing, whose books I used to carry around with me, until I saw him on *The Late Late Show*, when he turned out to be no more or less perceptive than any of the intoxicated Scotsmen I'd encountered in the RIE. In the end, despite my reservations about his speciality, I went to see Professor Clare in Dublin on a couple of occasions in the summer of 2007. He'd been one of those many famous UCD L&H debaters who go on to be popular public figures. The only thing that surprised me about him was that he was smaller than I had expected and, with his then 'Dubliners'-style beard, he looked remarkably like Oonagh Hayes's husband, Jarlath, another man for whom I had much time.

Professor Clare was soft-spoken, polite and non-judgemental. He seemed a little world-weary, but was profoundly sympathetic to my plight, and he said that he recognised most of the themes and tropes in my account of myself, particularly those involving an over-busy physician. I really warmed to him, and he reminded me of mentors like Niall O'Donohoe, Brian Maurer and John Fennell, who had been so encouraging to me over the years. In retrospect, I think my own burnout was really coming to a head in 2007, the year I started to see the great psychiatrist for my 'melancholic mood'. It is clear from re-reading my various missives to the press that that was the year I also began to lose my sense of humour and started to develop a serious 'irony deficiency' myself. All my letters seem to be about the heartbreak of medical staffing issues, the political machinations around ED overcrowding, or the public health aspects of homicidal violence in Ireland, especially that driven by drug consumption, which many in the commentariat decline to see.

I was particularly – viscerally – exercised by the cocaine-fuelled 2006 shooting of 22-year-old mother Donna Cleary in Coolock, the savage 2008 killings in Drimnagh of two young Poles, Pawel Kalite and Marius Szwaijkos, both expertly skewered in the head with a screwdriver by a teenager high on alcohol, cannabis and pills, and the abduction, gang rape and murder of Marioara Rostas, an 18-year-old Romanian girl in Dublin in 2008. I wrote at length and with passion about these cases in letters and opinion pieces because I felt they were spectacular examples of the sort of public health threat represented by drug- or drink-induced impulsivity. I was, of course, acquainted with industrial amounts of human misery and horror. Coincidentally, just days before I returned to see Anthony Clare for a review of my mental state, my workplace was full of the stuff of potential nightmares. It was my weekend on-call, and I was called in half-a-dozen times to deal with a mixture of the usual and the increasingly usual. These included a young man who was fatally stabbed early on the Saturday morning, an elderly man who was clearly beyond resuscitation but whose family wanted us to keep 'working' on him, and a toddler who fell to her death from a second-storey window in a city-centre building near the Mercy. In total, I spent about twelve hours on the shopfloor, grappling with the fatal cases and their aftermath, but it was the belligerently intoxicated patients in the CDU, the victims of one man's crazy driving on a local road, and the 'fast-tracking' ambulatory patients which required the most time. Oddly, while the work was tiring, dispiriting and a little exasperating, what upset me most that weekend was hearing about two murders in Liverpool: the shooting of a nightclub doorman and an eleven-year-old boy in a park.

So when I went to see Professor Clare a couple of days later, I could offer him two basic reasons for the dejection he'd seen me with a few weeks previously, and for which he had suggested some antidepressant medication. Clearly, there was the personal round-the-clock battles within the hectic environment of Cork's emergency departments, with its countless distressed and sometimes critically ill and injured patients. But there was also the less personal but bigger picture of ever-expanding numbers of drug-fuelled murders and general savagery, about which I had been exercised for years. In truth, I didn't go into either category of explanation, as they really only amounted to 'more of the same', as far as I was concerned. And the kindly psychiatrist knew that. We touched briefly on counselling, and I think I made it clear that my preference was to not take antidepressant medication, if possible. And that really left just the elephant in the room, with which we were both very familiar: burnout.

I readily admit that I hadn't really delved into the subject of burnout back in 2007. Nor was it as clearly defined as it later became. So, while we skirted around the subject, it seemed to me that Clare was suggesting that it was an almost inescapable side-effect of being a doctor, especially one who was 'an officer in the trenches', and that my extracurricular work was only likely to make matters worse, even if he – of all people – appreciated that contributing to the media was something I felt was essential if the conditions and challenges within the emergency departments of the country were to be understood and addressed. The ultimate irony was that Anthony Clare's example – in his efforts over decades to promote a public understanding of his own speciality – was one of the reasons I felt compelled to do the same for emergency medicine.

So there remained the obvious question: what was I to do with that elephant in the room – burnout? And in the same way as it must be nigh-impossible (unless you're a genuine *mahout*, or elephant rider) to single-handedly push an elephant out of that imaginary room, I think the professor and I both knew that the burnout, as enormous a problem as it clearly was for me, and so many others, was just 'part of the job'. He and I were of similar scholastic and philosophical stock, having gone to comparable Catholic schools near Donnybrook. So guilt, stoicism and soldiering-on were all part of the gig. And I think he believed that I wasn't 'psychiatrically' unwell, but rather spiritually sickened by my occupational burden. I will never know, but I cannot imagine that he would have advised me to *abandon* medicine as a career, even if that were the 'cure'. Equally, I cannot imagine that I would have taken such advice, at the time, given that being a medic was what I did, it was what I felt compelled to do, and it was undoubtedly my *vocation*. No, whatever about medication that seemed to be worse-than-useless for me anyway, and whatever about potentially helpful counselling, I wouldn't be retiring any time soon.

I was really looking forward to seeing Professor Clare again after our last meeting, at the end of August 2007. In truth, the sessions with him provided the 'talking therapy' of which we often hear nowadays. But sadly, it wasn't to be. Ireland's most renowned psychiatrist died suddenly, at the age of just 64, on a visit to Paris several weeks later. I remember feeling rather selfishly grief-stricken, as if I'd lost a recently discovered, highly charismatic uncle. However, it seemed also like a sign to get back to work and stop moaning. After all, I was still very much alive.

Once More Unto the Breach

Oscar Wilde was right, as usual. 'True friends stab you in the front,' he remarked memorably. And I can vouch for this from personal experience. I think I was about twenty years old when my friend, David O'Donohoe, then a law student in UCD, delivered one of his more controversial verdicts. On this occasion, it was about my choice of career. 'The problem with medics, Chris,' he observed, shaking his handsome head sympathetically, in the manner of the superstar lawyer he was to become, 'is that they're *always* moaning.' A trivial enough barb, one might think, but the problem for me was that David's father, Niall, distinguished Professor of Paediatrics at Trinity College Dublin, brilliant paediatric neurologist and author of a world-famous textbook on childhood epilepsy, was actually my own emerging role model. In hearing his son's opinion, I experienced a significant degree of cognitive dissonance, that unpleasant mental conflict between what you hear and what you *want* to hear.

I have seldom known David to get such judgements wrong. In fact, his unfailing correctness and accompanying charm could easily be infuriating, if we weren't lifelong friends. Or very expensive, if I were his client. And now, decades later, I have to admit that David was spot-on. Medics do moan, mutter and gripe a great deal about the many crosses they have to bear. I know, because I've spent much of the past 40 years privately railing against the injustices of medical training and career prospects, and I've done my best publicly, on air or in the Letters pages, to politely protest about this and that problem in the EDs of these islands, or sometimes just about the burden of being a hospital consultant. In fact, way back, when I could still laugh, my letter to the *Irish Times* in April 2007 on that very subject achieved the coveted top spot, with my comment: 'Vilification of Irish hospital consultants regularly gets me humming my children's favourite ditty: "Nobody loves me, everybody hates me, think I'll go and eat worms".'

And my 2005 piece in *Medicine Weekly* blamed the problem of unhappy doctors on a simple mismatch between their ambitions and the reality of working in the Irish health service. In setting out my remedy – and I must issue an irony alert here – I urged medical readers to replace the behavioural 'vices' that tended to underlie their misery, like altruism, perfectionism and stoicism, with a little 'Groucho-Marxism', as I called it. In short, I suggested that doctors could learn to intone Groucho's perennially useful dictum: 'These are my principles. If you don't like 'em, I have others'. And yes, I was being both cynical *and* sarcastic.

Setting aside the very personal disappointment at 'losing' Professor Clare, or rather a potentially therapeutic relationship with him, I soon reverted to type and got back to work. In truth, I was pretty sure that he would have encouraged me to continue working, but to 'reflect' a bit more and 'adapt'. So I did, insofar as I tried to accommodate the workload of the EDs at CUH and the Mercy, and otherwise waited to see what turned up. I continued my personal mission to contribute to the public debate on ED overcrowding, medical staffing and drug-related violence. But I did have other interests, especially around the idea of the emergency department as 'public health observatory'.

Accordingly, I was particularly chuffed to be invited to Galway in 2007 to develop that idea. I've always loved Galway. Even before 1973, when I visited the City of the Tribes en route to Irish College in Connemara, I'd stayed there a few times with my mother. It wasn't just the compact feel of the place or the fresh Atlantic air that was so appealing, it just seemed like a purer, less metropolitan Ireland, exemplified by the Claddagh shawlies, the work of Garry Hynes and Mick Lally in the Druid Theatre and the odd story-filled lunch with my vivacious 'aunt-in-law' Pat O'Connell, historian and librarian at University College Galway, as it then was.

The invitation was to give a lecture at the First International Conference on Reducing Environmental Risks and Protecting Health, hosted by the HSE, the Environmental Health Department in Galway and UCG. It was a real honour to be asked to share a stage with leading Irish, British and American academics, representatives of the WHO and Health Protection Agency in England, and Duncan Stewart, the TV presenter and long-time environmental activist. And one of the highlights of the trip was strolling to the conference dinner venue through the city's Latin Quarter, and seeing so many students crowd affectionately around Duncan, who was clearly something of an Attenborough among the young people of Ireland.

My lecture was entitled, 'An Inconvenient Truth? The Emergency Department as Environmental Observatory' (borrowed shamelessly from the surprise hit movie of 2006, featuring former American Vice President Al Gore's slide show, which he'd shown over a thousand times to audiences worldwide). My own talk featured slides that I too had shown around the UK, Ireland and Europe, albeit a lot less often, and they illustrated my argument that the ED should not just be a repository for all of society's ills but could also be a 'lookout tower' for those same troubles. I outlined the surprising variety of environmental health emergencies seen in hospitals, from altitude illness to insect and reptile bites, lightning injuries to heat exhaustion, weird viral diseases to familiar food poisonings, and I suggested that climate change would probably increase the number of such threats.

I cited tragic examples of emergencies from that very week, including a hundred deaths in a Russian coal mine, the death of a young mother in a crash on the fog-bound M7 in Kildare, and recurrent *E. coli* contamination of the water in Galway. And I said that EDs globally had been passively and actively engaged with environmental issues like nightclub medicine, overdoses, violence, foot and mouth disease, *E. coli* cases, and the 2003 SARS outbreak in Toronto and the Far East. I readily acknowledged the 'inconvenience' of collecting data around threats like *E. coli*, violence and occupational injuries, but pointed out that *mapping* threats, such as where assaults, infections or occupational illnesses occur, was a crucial first step towards prevention. Cholera had been the most famous example of using maps to eradicate disease in the nineteenth century, and I argued that the cost of *not* fully understanding environmental hazards in Ireland included deaths in quarries and on foggy roads and trawlers, the closure of licensed premises and food outlets, EU fines for illegal water contamination and the scandals then associated with MRSA (of which Cork hospitals had the highest levels in Ireland in March 2007).

I mentioned that trawlers and quarries were among the most dangerous workplaces in Ireland, with about four individuals losing their lives annually in the related occupations. But in fact, the Irish Association for Emergency Medicine (IAEM) regularly pointed out that over 300 patients could be dying annually in Irish EDs due to overcrowding, because the numbers, noise and cramped conditions mean that medical deterioration or distress may sometimes not be spotted. Driving back from the West after the conference, it suddenly occurred to me that EDs are, in theory, some of the most hazardous environments in Ireland, for very sick people anyway.

That grim statistic and my lived experience explain why 'barbaric bedlam' was the description I used throughout 2007 to describe the conditions in both emergency departments in Cork, in plaintive letters to the management of both hospitals, to colleagues, to the media and in my own journal. Translated, this meant that there might be three or four times the number of patients that an ED was designed to accommodate on trolleys, so corridors were lined with trolleys literally as far as the eye could see. To put it at its simplest, both EDs in Cork were routinely 'bursting'. However, several tactical difficulties arose in addressing the grotesque overcrowding. First was the Confucian concept I'd learned as a trainee in Edinburgh, which I paraphrase as: 'to hear is to forget, to see is to recall, to do is to understand'. So only those working within EDs really grasp the problem.

Second, there was the bleak political fact that, while a quarter of the population of Ireland visits an ED every year, the experience is often so awful *or* so shockingly uneventful that people develop a kind of 'amnesia' when it comes to the next general election.

And third, while George Orwell famously said that restating the obvious was the first duty of intelligent people, the Minister for Health in 2007, Mary Harney, had herself declared a year earlier that the chronic overcrowding in EDs in the country was to be treated as a 'national emergency'. She asserted that 'every resource would be prioritised, and every action needed' would be taken to improve care for patients in EDs. And she added, 'People who need to be admitted will have beds, not trolleys, and the basics for human dignity. This will be put in place in the coming months. Anything less than this is not acceptable to the public, not acceptable to me, and not acceptable to the HSE.'

And so the situation stayed, more-or-less unremedied, for the rest of my hospital career. The Minister had accepted that the situation was of crisis proportions, and that something must and would be done. There was no argument. And then the next phase began. A task force was established to deal with the problem and its chair, Angela Fitzgerald, said that its aim was that no ED patient should wait to be admitted to a ward for more than six hours after assessment. And that was that, really. For the next few years, from my perspective, there ensued a fractious political period characterised by deployment of PR spin tactics, with most of the action involving refutation of the other side's numbers or disputation of what 'assessment' meant.

What actually happened on the healthcare frontline during 2007, and over the next four years, was that ED conditions got steadily worse, and people like me and Steve Cusack wrote increasingly irate and despairing letters to managers, colleagues and the press, pleading for help to overcome the bedlam, and the causes of the bedlam. We pleaded with in-house colleagues to stop telling their patients to 'pop back to A&E if you have a problem after …' surgery, chemo, scope or whatever. We appealed to GPs not to send us longstanding cases for second opinions, x-rays or scans, because of lengthy outpatient waiting lists. I even wrote an open letter to Irish medical graduates, imploring them to stay in Ireland to help in the trenches before they headed off to sunnier and money-er climes.

In addition, notwithstanding the gratifying success of my non-clinical work introducing the annual Final MB Clinical Skills Course in UCC and reviving the weekly Intern Teaching Programme and Grand Rounds at CUH, I had resigned from my role as Director of Postgraduate Medical Education there because it was eating into my clinical time in two besieged EDs. I also reduced my involvement in Club Cork, the staff training programme in the city's pubs and clubs, which was another satisfying extracurricular initiative that I could no longer justify, although I was able to hand over the baton to a very worthy successor, the former CUH Intern, Conor Deasy.

Meanwhile, the politicians and their PR people were referring endlessly to the work of the task force, and the media spotlight shifted to the issue of the hospital consultants' new contract, which Minister Harney planned to push through, regardless of the failure of the NHS version that preceded and informed it. Not long after I returned from Galway to the purgatorial environment of Cork's EDs, the government was rewarded with 'manna from heaven' when a consultant anaesthetist described the proposed salary of €250,000 for consultants agreeing to the new deal as a 'Mickey Mouse' offer that would not attract Irish-trained doctors back from America, where they could easily earn salaries of $500,000.

The media understandably lapped this up and the late, great Mary Raftery, one of Ireland's most estimable journalists (and in the year above me at school), wrote a piece in the *Irish Times*, on 19 April 2007, full of righteous anger at greedy and bumptious consultants. As it happened, I generally agreed with Mary, not least because I've always been primarily a public system doctor with an unusually modest private practice. I recognise that there will always be a wide variation in medical salaries, but I sometimes despair at the few egregiously avaricious consultants in the ranks. So I wrote a letter to the *Irish Times*, perhaps trying to defend the indefensible. I explained that the perceived power, affluence and hubris of Irish consultants stemmed from their scarcity, the brutality of their training and the bureaucracy in which they were daily mired. And I argued that the real solution was primarily economic: their numbers needed to be increased, as did the extraordinary training and resources they needed to do their highly specialised work.

I argued that the Minister's preferred solution – a hastily imposed, hyper-regulatory new contract and Medical Practitioners' Bill – was the riskiest political interference in the Irish health service since its inception, and that it vividly illuminated her conviction that *consultants* were a root cause of the bed shortages, cancelled operations, missing outpatient slots and sluggish reform of the health service. But it was based on prejudice, I said, and Ireland actually depended on a tiny number of overworked, overpaid and outspoken consultants doing the jobs of umpteen counterparts abroad. I then offered my usual diagnostic suggestion, that the Minister and her department learn from the mistakes recently made in the UK, where a smear campaign against consultants, depicting them as untrustworthy plutocrats, had resulted in a collapse in seniors doctors' confidence, leadership and productivity.

Even now, in 2021, I stick by what I wrote in that letter, along with my conclusion, that *doctors really do tend to speak the truth*. Only now, there is also plenty of evidence that the contract that was imposed in 2008 was pretty disastrous, at least if you consider the current hospital waiting lists and 700 consultant vacancies in the Irish health service to be far from ideal.

Despite the loud silence that usually rewarded my utterances, I kept fighting the good fight. I spent the rest of 2007 on 'a one-man A&E campaign' – as my favourite medical politician, Christine O'Malley, then President of the Irish Medical Organisation, sympathetically dubbed it. My absolute top priority was moving the ED at the Mercy Hospital, in Cork's city centre, from a couple of rooms in a corner of the old building to a purpose-built, state-of-the-art facility in the modern block across the road. This meant months of pleading with management about the need to end the squalor in the old department and reminding them that there were often over twenty patients waiting to be admitted in a six-trolley unit, while levels of aggression and violence towards the staff and other patients had become really frightening. The fact that a new ED at CUH had been opened by Minister Harney in 2005 was a particular spur to me, as I'd experienced for myself the benefit to both service and staff morale that a new, purpose-built department could provide, at least for a while.

In his defence, the Mercy's Chief Executive Officer, Pat Madden, was profoundly sympathetic. After all, he'd driven the construction of the new €4.7 million department (in whose design I had been involved, with Anne O'Keeffe, the ED's pioneering Advanced Nurse Practitioner). The problem was that the hospital just didn't have the funding from Dublin to open the new enlarged department and to employ the necessary number of extra nurses and ancillary staff. I hope that, in hindsight, Pat and others in management can understand why staff like me spoke to the local press, urging 'the powers that be' to do everything they could to open the new department (which in the end lay idle for twenty months, while the warranty on new equipment within it ran out). After all, difficulty makes people difficult.

I also hope that Ms Harney will understand how upset the Mercy ED staff were when she accused them of 'holding the government to ransom' over the opening of the new facility. As Mary Dunnion, Director of Nursing at the Mercy, explained in the *Irish Examiner* on 13 August 2008, the staff were desperate to move into the new facility, and she stoutly defended them, saying that experts had agreed that moving into a new department with a much bigger footprint and far more rooms required a substantial increase in staffing. It seems remarkable now that anyone would suggest that the same number of staff could manage a near-doubling of patient numbers in an era of enormous complexity and rapidly advancing care. I think the Mercy ED sees about 15,000 more patients annually than it did after I first arrived in 1999, when it comprised two or three rooms.

Another political project in which I found myself engaged was the Doctors' Alliance. This was a short-lived network of medics anxious to promote the public health service, who wanted to counter the stream of grim news and win back the faith of the public.

I was invited to one particularly animated meeting in a Dublin hotel, at which I had the pleasure of renewing old friendships with Orla Hardiman, Professor of Neurology at TCD and a UCD classmate, and Brian Maurer, my former boss and mentor at St Vincent's. The assembled doctors were mostly concerned with the decline in staff morale, the lack of a measured public debate about the purpose and capacity of the health service and, above all, pursuing what was right for patients. It was a really hopeful moment, but sadly the noble project petered out, mostly ignored by the HSE and Department of Health, which blamed much of the bad news on doctors going to the press.

Personally, I thought the despondency in the media about our health service mostly reflected the dreary public wrangling over the new contract between the Minster and her representatives and the Irish Hospital Consultants' Association. There was also the first of several scandals to affect the relatively new HSE (set up in 2005), over the misdiagnosis of breast cancer at Portlaoise Hospital, and the eight-year-long waiting lists to see some specialists. Alas, one of the problems with well-meaning lobbyists (like me, the Doctors' Alliance, and sundry others) is that we sometimes step on each other's toes. So I was also moved to defend myself in the *Irish Times*, in November 2007, against a bizarre assertion by Marie O'Connor, author of *Emergency: Irish Hospitals in Chaos*, that EDs had been satisfactorily run by general surgeons and physicians until these were replaced by 'arcane subspecialists', like yours truly, as part of an evolving 'empire' of emergency care.

It is worth bearing in mind that even though I kept restating the obvious, the overcrowding in the country's EDs wasn't becoming any less or any easier to deal with. The reality is that when the waiting room, the ambulance bay, the Resus Room, and every other part of an emergency department is occupied with sick or distressed or deranged people, the atmosphere can be frightening for everyone. And because most patients on trolleys have one or two companions with them, the congestion resembles a match day outside Lansdowne Road or Croke Park. It is hard to push through the throng, never mind deliver dignified, thoughtful care. And very often, it is hard to find a single private space to undertake an intimate examination of a patient. Inevitably mishaps occur, like elderly patients falling off trolleys and sustaining serious injuries like hip fractures. And in the waiting room, where often people have to stand for hours, it is commonplace to have fights between patients or relatives, with or without the involvement of security staff. Needless to add, with people waiting for hours and hours, the reception and nursing staff often 'get it in the neck'.

And meanwhile the serious emergency care is squeezed in, like the critical care in the Resus Room for those with life-threatening heart attacks, cardiac arrest, respiratory or liver failure, severe injury or overdose. Or the infusions of medication or fluids to patients on trolleys. Or the urinary catheterisation of a patient in terrible pain just behind a curtain which is the only thing separating him from the screaming elderly lady on the next trolley with her painful hip fracture. The stitching and plastering sometimes must be done in just one dedicated cubicle, which becomes the Minors area for the 70-odd percent of patients who walk in and out each day.

And, as if that isn't bad enough, every so often a particularly deranged and violent patient will suddenly arrive in the back of an ambulance, surrounded by paramedics, guards and security staff, and occasionally handcuffed to the side of the trolley because they are trying to bite, headbutt or punch the professionals. These patients can bring added fear and chaos into a packed ED, as they struggle deliriously on the trolley. Usually, the cause is a stimulant drug like cocaine, one of the weirder headshop-type powders or new psychoactive substances, or synthetic cannabinoids like 'Spice', and while the treatment is mainly about sedation, the patients can be profoundly mentally deranged for days, or longer, and sudden death is not uncommon, particularly with cocaine.

There were some deaths widely reported in the news that really affected me in 2007, like that of 14-year-old Michelle Bray from Dungarvan, a 'troubled teen' who died after sniffing the contents of a deodorant can. Her case prompted me to get involved in a public health awareness initiative in Cork around VSA, or volatile substance abuse. Often called 'the forgotten drug epidemic', it periodically kills 11–13-year-olds, for whom sniffing glue, butane or anti-perspirant is often the first high. Another Dungarvan native, Niall O'Riordan, died in Dublin in July after taking ecstasy and cocaine. The latter drug also killed three young people in quick succession at the end of 2007. Two of them, John Grey and Kevin Doyle, were from Waterford, while the third was Katy French, from Stillorgan, one of Ireland's best-known socialites. The result was what criminologists call a 'moral panic', or a collective outpouring of anguish about the sudden, devastating tragedies. But cocaine had worried me for years, and I'd fretted publicly since the 1990s about its worst side-effects: extreme violence and sudden death.

As always, the difficulty in conducting a so-called 'honest debate' about the issue of drug consumption in Ireland lies in the scarcity of up-to-date local data, but whenever serious surveys are undertaken, the trajectory in terms of hard drug consumption does almost always seem to be heading upwards. For instance, the Health Research Board published figures in early July 2021 suggesting a six-fold increase in the number of young women consuming cocaine in this country over the past five years or so, and added that the range of hazardous drugs now being consumed by all sexes is widening relentlessly. The European Monitoring Centre for Drugs and Drug Addiction (EMCDDA) Report of 2020 said that 'the most notable trend [in Irish drug use] is the continued increase in the number of cases presenting for treatment for problem cocaine use. Numbers of first-time entrants [for treatment] reporting cocaine as their primary drug … reached its highest level in 10 years in 2017.' Ten years before that was 2007, a year when I was especially vocal about cocaine-related deaths and violence. The same source was quoted as saying that 7.8 per cent of certain age groups in Ireland had taken cocaine in their lifetime. And it was the EMCDDA which stated that Ireland had the third-highest cocaine usage in Europe, just behind Spain and the UK, where over 10 per cent of younger people had taken cocaine at some stage. As always, I defer to higher authority in such matters.

For instance, the EMCDDA in Lisbon employs a reputable group of scientists and the scale of cocaine usage in Ireland that they describe is serious. I'm inclined to say of all drugs that the *rate* of drug-related health issues (like critical illness or death) only 'really' matters if the *denominator* is big. The ED rule of thumb is that about 10 per cent of users of drugs like cannabis and cocaine run into genuinely serious issues. To me, 10 per cent of 10 per cent of a country's young adult population looks like a substantial problem but, in the absence of the resources needed to capture good data on violence, drink- and drug-related conditions seen in Irish EDs, the public must rely on reports from people like me. It doesn't mean that they have to like *my* version of honesty, although I, for one, would love a public debate about drugs in which people could disagree without being disagreeable.

The following year, 2008, saw more of the same preoccupations. In February, I wrote of the Mercy ED: 'it is not unusual to have 22 patients on trolleys for prolonged periods in a tiny, cramped unit with 6 trolley spaces, which has one patient toilet (a sluice room) and two staff sinks, one of which is often inaccessible because of the trolleys. The conditions are deplorable, frightening and driving dedicated staff to despair (and resignation).' Lamentably, that remained my message until December when, after twenty months of waiting, the new department opened. Finally, I got to share a small office with Bernice, the long-suffering ED secretary at the Mercy, which was not a windowless ex-storeroom, but had shelves and a window. At last, I didn't have to twist my entire torso to use the computer.

The department itself was so (relatively) wonderful that I was proud to show it to visitors, like Professor Brendan Drumm, then head of the HSE, and to explain that we now had a facility that was co-designed by the staff to stream critically ill, trolley-bound and walking patients separately. It also gave me considerable satisfaction that, after years of pleading with the management, the new unit even had a staff room, an eleventh-hour concession. Astonishingly, I had to beg for a space where nurses and doctors could grab a cup of tea and a sandwich in between seeing patients.

I was still not happy with Minister Harney, though, after her earlier veiled threats to the Mercy staff, and I was moved to write to the *Sunday Business Post*, this time in November 2007, when Aileen O'Meara wrote that 'while there may still be occasional chaotic scenes in (Irish) hospitals, especially during winter, in general the problem has been tackled'. I described this as an 'Orwellian piece of fiction' and suggested that even a cub reporter could have ascertained the reality of constant ED overcrowding by visiting their nearest hospital. And I pointed out that, with the global economic downturn of 2008, this wasn't merely a matter of dinner-party debate but was of importance to anyone who couldn't afford to use the new private urgent care facilities proliferating in the country, which were very much part of Ms Harney's vision for the future of Irish healthcare.

The overcrowding in both EDs in Cork (and everywhere else) worsened relentlessly, so my one-man campaign continued in other preventive directions. I contributed to an educational video on alcohol misuse driven by the Alcohol Liaison Nurse at CUH and based on the alcohol-related caseload in the CDU there. And exchanging hats, I gave a talk to the Irish Hospitality Industry's Exhibition at the RDS, where I extolled the joys of a well-run pub and urged publicans to diversify their activities into good food, posh coffee and interesting non-alcoholic drinks. I spoke at a conference in Cork for GPs on the relationship between alcohol and drugs and suicide. But the most haunting insight at that meeting came from a chilling account of a son's sudden suicide in New York by his eloquent, heartbroken mother. She told the audience how her talented offspring had been getting ready to go out for the night with his friends and, just as they all were heading down to the taxi, one of them had come back (possibly even his sister) to hurry him up, only to find he had just hanged himself in the hallway. The frightening conclusion was that such tragedies sometimes seem so *impulsive*.

Ongoing trends on the Cork EDs' observatory radar in 2008 included the growing number of cases of poisoning with BZP, a headshop drug, and again I was struck by the death in Derby of a 12-year-old boy due to inhaling deodorant fumes. In the UK, it was reported that official violence statistics might not be as reliable as those found in ED records. Yet again, I wrote about the importance of recognising the 'lookout tower' role of the ED in such statistics.

I had still been involved with 'Club Health' since my Liverpool days, and in 2008 I attended the annual conference in Ibiza, where almost all the issues we had described at the first conference in Cream in 1997 were now standard fare, such as hearing damage in DJs, the environmental hazards in and around clubs globally, and the epidemiology of newer synthetic drugs.

The most fascinating aspect of that Balearic trip was visiting giant nightclubs, like Manumission and Pacha. It would take a large coffee-table book to adequately describe these spectacular pleasure domes, which could accommodate 10,000 clubbers on a single night. They were as far as one could imagine from the cramped Harcourt Street and Leeson Street clubs of my youth. However, one thing remained essentially unchanged from the 1990s and the 1970s. A bottle of water there cost about €10, which meant that while Club Health had made some progress around the world since 1997, it had a long way to go in terms of customer care in those hot, sweaty and breathtakingly profitable fleshpots.

The subject of drug- and drink-related violence continued to generate headlines, and in 2009 I was invited on to *The Late Late Show* to discuss it with my friend, RTÉ reporter and author Brian O'Connell. He was even more apprehensive and dry-mouthed than me going up the steps behind the famous stage, until – wordlessly – I offered him a 'pill' to ease his nerves. We went on, the cameras rolled, and sure enough, Brian was as cool as a cucumber throughout. Afterwards, when he asked me what my 'homeopathic rescue remedy' was, I confessed that it was a peppermint TicTac. We both roared laughing at the beauty of *belief*. Or Big Placebo.

The trends in 2009 were good and bad. The number of road traffic deaths in the country was at an all-time low, but the levels of violence everywhere were really distressing. Sadly, in Cork, in spite of my talk about 'mapping', my colleagues in the ambulance service and I were so busy that we couldn't record *precisely* where assaults were happening in the city, although we had a reasonable idea. That was a pity. So, too, was the multiplicity of big drug seizures nationally, several heroin deaths in Cork and the first death I'd encountered from 'crystal meth', a frightening drug that has caused devastation throughout the USA but is thankfully still uncommon here.

Just as worrying was the surge in use of headshop drugs like Mephedrone, or 'Meow Meow', which was causing me huge concern as it tended to affect teenagers mostly and seemed to cause shocking levels of prolonged delirium, psychosis and associated violence (for instance, a teenage girl threatening her mother in the north inner city with a kitchen knife). The effect on the existing levels of misery in the bursting Mercy ED was particularly upsetting, as the addled teens were a nightmare to manage.

The two EDs were perpetually swamped in 2009, but I was becoming equally frustrated by the difficulty in recruiting young doctors. That year we had been reaching as far east as Moldova and Belorussia, but we were still finding it nigh-impossible to get enough doctors to work even briefly in the trenches. I was spending hours popping back and forth to HR to interview candidates on the phone, or in person, with little success. I was also exasperated by what I perceived as the dwindling productivity of some junior doctors, particularly those who had never worked in Ireland before, who had been trained in a different system and spoke English as a second language. Some of them seemed to have no idea about the Irish version of emergency medicine and occasionally seemed to 'see' but not really 'manage' two or three patients over an eight-hour shift. One of my suggested remedies was to bring in a few local Interns and more Advanced Nurse Practitioners (ANPs) to treat walking patients in every ED, under the supervision of a consultant. I was already working with brilliant ANPs in both departments, and we'd had Interns working in the ED at CUH for years, so I was convinced that some progress was possible in that general direction. Moreover, as a former Intern tutor, I was well aware that some medical graduates in Ireland couldn't actually obtain Intern posts, so this seemed like a perfect way to address that scandalous mismatch (in which medical training of overseas medical students in Ireland was essentially incomplete).

Sadly, in my growing desperation, I went on and on (and on) to my consultant colleagues about the possibility of replacing a cohort of 'unreliable or unwilling' medics with ANPs and local first-year graduates, but I did so to the extent that we eventually fell out. *Mea culpa.* I freely admit that I can be *intense* when it comes to some issues. Irritatingly intense, sometimes. And, occasionally, intensely irritating. This was one such example, and I regret it, but I still believe that more ANPs and more Interns in EDs would help. And I am pleased to say that, despite the disagreements of 2009, there are now ANPs and Interns in many EDs around the country, doing wonderful work.

In early 2010, as a sort of therapeutic exercise, I compiled a list of all my 'Big Ideas' for a radical reconfiguration of the way EDs might be organised, at least in Cork. My primary idea was that electronic technology should be used where possible, like e-learning, e-board rounds, e-appointments for GP rapid access clinics, and e-follow-up, along with texting patients when their test results were back. I thought we should separate ambulatory care completely from trolley-bound cases, and I thought that first aid should be made more easily available at pharmacies.

I continued to suggest that 'scribes', or assistants who take notes, would be hugely helpful for busy doctors (as they are in the USA), and I noted that medical recruitment at the time was so difficult and often so fruitless that we should move away from recruiting short-term medical staff and move towards longer contracts. Finally, I suggested that doctors' work rate in the ED should be monitored (the number of patients they saw per shift) and this should go into their references. None of this thinking would have come as a surprise to anyone in business, and most of the ideas came from reading about management in the weekend newspapers, but I was to learn very painfully that such *revolutionary* thinking could be perceived, in some parts, as profoundly dangerous.

I also contacted some of the leading GPs in Cork to plead with them for help addressing certain referrals. Recent, exasperating examples had included a child with a lifelong eye condition who waited for hours in the Mercy ED (where there was no eye service), and a patient with a six-month history of warts on their feet. I told them that the EDs were in a state of 'meltdown' for want of staff, beds and space. Arguably the top GP trainer in Cork wrote back to say that he had witnessed the chaos personally, so I was 'speaking to the converted'. In fact, I wrote to quite a few friendly GPs at the time, to convey my anguish about non-urgent cases arriving into the bedlam in the EDs, only to wait for six to ten hours before being told they were in the wrong place. But the low point was when I phoned one GP about a similar case, and he told me that he would continue to refer patients wherever and whenever he 'f—ing wanted'. That was my last such courtesy call.

Meanwhile, the medical staffing crisis was getting so bad that I penned an opinion piece in the *Irish Times* on 2 July 2010 called, 'Devising A Treatment Plan For An Understaffed System'. This was primarily about the need for the Irish health service to get away from its strategically disastrous reliance on a fickle supply of overseas doctors, to replace those we'd trained but who declined to work at the frontline. I again enthused about the employment of more Interns and ANPs. And I proposed a sort of community service for our medical graduates in return for their training, as is seen in so many other parts of the world. Alas, I made the grave mistake of using a word I'd found on Dr Google, to describe 'a legal agreement or contract'. I deliberately used the word in relation to getting some would-be medical students to sign up to a six- to twelve-month stint at the health service frontline in return for a waiving of the controversial HPAT entrance test. That word was 'indenture', and it was a sign of my age and my very old-fashioned use of language that I forgot its other non-legal, political meanings. That poor choice of words was to haunt me for years, as the notion of 'indentured servitude' from our unhappy colonial past was continuously brought up by my detractors.

In addition to our normal heavy ED workload, there was an ever-worsening situation with headshop drugs in Cork, and a growing number of delirious and violent youngsters arriving in the EDs. So again, I took to the newspapers, and I wrote an opinion piece in the *Irish Examiner* on 18 January 2010, entitled, 'We Need Our Headshops Examined'. In it, I deplored so-called legal highs, sold freely all around Cork and the rest of the Republic by then, and referred to four ambulance cases related to the products over the previous weekend.

It may sound like I was firing off all these letters and opinion pieces into an indifferent void, just for fun, but every now and then something I said struck a chord, making it all worthwhile. In fact, I received two highly unexpected political plaudits in 2010. The first, ironically, was from the

Minister for Health herself, Deputy Mary Harney, who in an Oireachtas debate on 3 February described yours truly as 'one of the leading emergency medical physicians in the country', noting that I had suggested that legislation, education and cultural change were required to tackle the growing scourge of headshops.

I don't know if she was unconsciously channelling my January article, but she said that anyone who spent €30 on 'bath salts' (as headshop drugs were deliberately mislabelled) needed their head examined. In fact, my article was referred to repeatedly in the debate, and I confess I was shocked but delighted that emergency legislation was introduced just a few months later, in May 2010. This effectively closed headshops in Ireland. It didn't drive the problem underground, as many predicted at the time, because the drugs had originally been purchased online, then sold in 'pop-up' headshops. But what it did do was to bring an abrupt end to the epidemic of headshop drugs driving a huge added ED and psychiatric burden nationally. And the respite for exhausted ED staff was extremely welcome.

The second plaudit came in a letter to the *Irish Examiner* on 18 June, entitled 'Man For Our Time', by Tom Fitzgerald in Limerick, who wanted me to run for the Dáil as a result of my efforts in relation to headshops. 'It is men like him our country needs in the corridors of power', he said, much too kindly.

Sadly, that was the last public support I was to receive for a long time, and any hubris I might have briefly experienced after all this political admiration was to evaporate in the following year, my *annus horribilis*.

Things Fall Apart

I suppose like many people in Ireland I felt I knew Gerry Ryan, the much-loved RTÉ presenter who died suddenly and tragically in April 2010. We'd actually been on nodding terms in the 1970s, when we were both young men about (Dublin) town, and I'm pretty sure he was at a raucous party in my house around 1978, although we'd never been in the same social circle. Still, after I found myself periodically chatting on his morning radio show in the Noughties, I came to enjoy his effervescence, quickfire conversation and mercurial temperament. He often referred to his 'partying' during the programme, and occasionally one would suspect that there'd been some consternation in Montrose when he arrived late for work and his eager waiting audience.

Nonetheless, Gerry's famous nocturnal social life didn't seem to detract from his capacity to entertain, inform and educate his legion of loyal listeners, and it was always a pleasure to converse with him about the issues of the hour. But I remember looking at him on TV in the year or two before he died and thinking to myself that he really was partying *much* too hard for a man of his age: he looked exhausted, flushed and overweight. And the last time we talked, months before he passed away, it dawned on me that he had actually been taking whatever I'd said before with a large pinch of salt. He'd more or less said so, when he'd told me that he used to believe I was 'so wound up' about cocaine that I needed a holiday, but now he was beginning to think I might have been right all along. That's how I remember it anyway: a sense of having almost persuaded him of the dangers. Almost.

Sadly, in hindsight, he had been neither convinced nor converted by what I'd been saying for years: a cocktail of cocaine and alcohol can be lethal due to the formation of a compound that seems to be peculiarly toxic to the heart, called coca-ethylene. Tragically, at the inquest, Gerry's death seemed to be a classic narrative of lethal cocaine poisoning: a hard-to-shake habit, a significant consumption of alcohol and, possibly, a fatal misjudgement that 'one line won't do any harm'. One thing borrows another. A few drinks, resistance is lowered, and the powder is easily available, so why not? But here's a brutal biological fact: for reasons we don't understand, even a single line of powdered cocaine taken by someone who has consumed the drug for years, and has done so without 'obvious' harm, can occasionally be lethal. Especially when there is an underlying condition. This was the case for Gerry, as the autopsy revealed a degree of myocarditis, or heart muscle inflammation, which is one of the markers, and hazards, of long-term cocaine consumption. Which left me asking: 'Will people never learn?' And then I pressed the accelerator on my own course to self-destruction.

I was certainly making misjudgements at this time. I had begun to succumb to the anger part of my burnout, along with chronic fatigue, cynicism and feeling under siege. I believed that many of my consultant and management colleagues thought I was always 'ranting' and 'attention-seeking', and they would certainly have had a point. Moreover, I was ignoring the physical impact of years of pressure.

And then I did something almost suicidally ill-judged, which was my experiment in impulsive outbursts live on the *Today with Pat Kenny* RTÉ radio programme, on 10 February 2011. A little like my panic attack at the surgeons' conference in Limerick ten years earlier, this time a purple mist descended as I prepared to rush off to deal with the Cork airport crash that morning. So when Pat invited me to offer an insight into the causes of the city's ED overcrowding, beyond the usual patients-on-trolleys stuff, I obliged. I brought up the issue of inappropriate GP referrals to bursting EDs. I was thinking of the really long-term cases, like warts, worn-out joints or people on waiting lists for scans. Then I mentioned the productivity of junior doctors, like the ones I'd observed that week seeing two, three or four patients in eight hours. And last, but by no means least, I talked of leadership by senior hospital managers. I referred to the fact that, in the UK, it was a government rule that ED patients needed to be discharged within about four hours of presentation or sanctions would be imposed on the managers. I suggested that healthcare leaders in Ireland needed to be more frequent visitors to their hospital's ED. These were all issues I'd been talking about for years, concerns that were consuming me, and which coalesced that day into what was an incendiary analysis of unbearable working conditions, which were the primary cause of my own rage and despair.

On all the issues, I was talking about 'facts', with considerable feeling. But what I failed to do was to remember that – in political terms – *feelings* can be more important than facts. Still steaming after I finished my brief but angry sermon, I left the Metropole Hotel and hurried back to CUH to help with the response to the major incident at the airport. And then, beginning to cool down, I headed to the Mercy to play my part in one of the busiest days ever seen in its ED, due to patients being diverted from its bigger sister hospital.

It wasn't until the following day that I experienced the full, fiery blast of outrage from my colleagues in general practice and doctors-in-training. The junior doctors were particularly angered by my use of the phrase, 'when I was a baby doctor', in relation to the number of patients young doctors used to see in a shift in my day. Again, it was an innocent slip of the tongue, employing a phrase that my medical peer group use in reminiscences, but it was seized upon as *proof* of my disdain for doctors-in-training.

The rage directed at me was initially filtered through a courteous 'covering' email from Professor Sean Tierney, President of the IMO, who I knew well as I was a member of the IMO's consultant committee, and we'd been on very friendly terms and quite closely aligned, I thought. Indeed, the last time we'd exchanged substantial emails was in 2010, when he supported my view that the outsourcing of Ireland's cervical smear testing to American laboratories that year was an egregious strategic and moral mistake.

Sean sent me a copy of the official IMO Statement to the *Today with Pat Kenny* show, regarding my contribution, in which he objected 'strongly' to what he called my 'crude and groundless criticisms' of my junior and senior colleagues and said that I had 'managed to tarnish the reputation of a generation of hard working doctors with some crass comments'. He suggested I was 'glorifying the good ol' days' of my youth and I seemed 'almost wistful for an era of chaotic hospitals which many of us will not remember fondly'. He concluded: 'The problem in the health service has not been created by lazy doctors or lazy nurses. It has been created by lazy thinking and soundbite explanations from those who think that there are simple solutions to complex problems.'

I must admit, I wasn't used to such 'collective' censure and it was certainly one of the most painful communications I'd ever received in my career. I also thought it was profoundly unfair towards someone who had spent so many years thinking about and trying to enhance the experience of patients and staff in different hospitals. The fact that Sean's immediate predecessor as IMO President, Neil Brennan, came to my defence in an emailed reply was of some comfort. He asked, 'Has Chris said anything that was actually untrue?' to which the gist of the response seemed to be: No, but what he said was offensive to many of his GP and junior colleagues.

In any case, I duly fell on my sword and resigned from the IMO consultant committee. I also enthusiastically endorsed my replacement on the committee, Peadar Gilligan, an immensely amiable and dynamic consultant in emergency medicine who went on to become the IMO President himself, not long after. It's an ill wind, as is so often remarked.

The official IMO reprimand was disconcerting enough, but what was much worse was the level of venom directed towards me by GPs in the Cork area, some of whom wrote to the CEO of CUH to complain, apparently demanding that I be disciplined. Judging by some of the letters and abusive phone calls I received, and the tirade of a formerly friendly GP on the side of the pitch at a rugby match, who roared that I'd *always* be 'the most hated consultant in Ireland', many of them would have gladly strung me up on the Wilton roundabout outside CUH.

Alongside this, there was the cohort of doctors-in-training who took to social media to denounce me in a Twitter pile-on that I was urged to avoid by the few remaining non-consultant doctors talking to me at work. Many doctors-in-training blanked me on hospital corridors, city streets and in shops for years afterwards. Although I was being quoted liberally in regard to the 'indenture' debate, I was effectively no-platformed and remained uninvited to meetings at which mandatory or negotiated stints at the healthcare frontline by trainees were debated that year.

This was despite the fact that I was singularly responsible for triggering the ongoing intense debate in the medical press. It was interesting that the *Irish Medical Times* suggested around half its readers were on 'my' side, and to see the debate spilling into the TV studios. Still, it was little consolation for someone who'd made a career out of being likeable. I don't exaggerate when I say that the contempt of my younger colleagues was the hardest thing I have ever had to contend with as a consultant.

As if the ostracism by much of the profession wasn't enough, I was summoned not long after my radio debacle to the Chief Executive's Office in CUH to account for myself, and my comments about GPs, 'in the context of my contract'. I was invited to bring a 'representative' with me, if I wished. I can assure those who think consultants are a thick-skinned, fat-cat elite that I am none of these things. Indeed, I would venture to say that I belong to the opposing thin-skinned tribe, and it was only the support of two top lawyers,

Gerald Moloney and David Pearson, that enabled me to get through a process that made me feel like my 14-year-old self, sweating in the school corridor, listening for the dreaded footsteps of the headmaster. In fact, the next half-decade felt as if I'd suddenly slid back down a very long snake into the anguish and uncertainty of the teen years, without the advantage of experience. It felt like a middle-age life crisis, with added responsibility, hostility and incivility.

My burnout, and the outburst stemming from it, didn't just send my career down in flames, it caused me a very great deal of pain. I'd become alienated from friends and colleagues, just as the Maslach Burnout Inventory would have predicted, and as I oscillated at speed between patients and departments in the few years after my 'cancelling', trying to do as much as I could, I found I just couldn't do my best anymore. Frankly, I felt too isolated, despondent and depleted of the enthusiasm for which I was once affectionately mocked. I occasionally imagine that if I hadn't had to endure the additional label of 'the most hated consultant in Ireland' for the final decade, I might have carried on. But I know the burnout would have eventually gotten to me.

And when I say 'gotten to me', I mean that I might have succumbed to ill-health or impulsive self-harm. Suffice it to say that I had frequent desperately dark moments.

The tragedy is that my life-threatening 'spiritual anaemia' was mostly work-related. Before my radio debacle, I had long been able to carry on regardless in the trench warfare of EDs in Cork, Liverpool and Edinburgh, but that was with the nourishing affection of patients and colleagues, particularly the medical trainees, nurses and permanent staff of the EDs. But with all the blackballing by so many younger graduates and GPs in 2011, the gaslighting by a few hospital colleagues, and my own physical health issues, I just didn't have the strength to go on.

At the start of the downward spiral, the conditions, staffing difficulties and bedlam in both EDs remained the same and over the weeks following the 2011 interview, I thought I was going to implode from stress. Thankfully, my darling wife prevented that from happening, along with my own brilliant GP, Dr Nuala O'Connor, and Professor John Gallagher, the particularly empathetic occupational health physician at CUH, who despatched me back to St John of God's Hospital in Dublin, a matter of yards from where I'd grown up. I wasn't there to be detained (the stuff of locals' bad dreams), but I was fortunate to see Professor Abbie Lane, one of Ireland's foremost psychiatrists in the area of occupational stress and bullying.

That was a piece of exceptional good fortune. It wasn't quite Bingo!, but I certainly felt as if I was in the right niche in the medical market, after my previous curtailed engagement with the late Anthony Clare. Professor Lane quickly recognised my occupational stressors and strains, she set out a plan of treatment and referred me for counselling, before discharging me back to Cork. And my most loyal old school friend, Peter Kenny, was there to take me for lunch afterwards, for a man-to-man debriefing. I cannot count the number of times in the past five decades when Peter has rung me to see how I am, just when I needed *someone* to be bothered, but couldn't bring myself to make that call. The same applied to another lifelong friend from Dalkey, Jack Fitzgerald, who has been the most constant and regular visitor from Dublin since the Lukes moved to Cork, and who always makes me laugh.

Truly, I count my blessings, which mainly take the form of enduring, life-affirming friendships.

My luck held. Over the following weeks, as I grappled with the usual chaos at work and the icy demeanour of those who still refused to engage with me, and reflected on the psychiatrist's advice to take time out, solicitous neighbours offered me the use of their holiday home in West Cork. In the end, I took six weeks off, my longest period of leave since the 1980s. For a fortnight anyway, I walked the beach in Inchydoney, read yarns from the Napoleonic era by my favourite author, Patrick O Brian, and wrote copiously in my journal. That break confirmed the truth of the WHO definition of burnout. It is a strictly *occupational* disease, caused by the stress of work and the workplace, and it is relieved by taking time away from both.

I was immensely gratified to find that the sea air, the solitude and the simple pleasures of walking, reading and listening to the radio were as satisfying as ever they'd been. Thankfully, I wasn't going mad, I didn't have endogenous depression, and I wasn't intrinsically melancholic.

What I fully appreciated was that my workload was toxic, as were my workplaces, but I also found that I really missed the core work, helping other people in crisis, for the weeks I was away. So, by May 2011, ready or not, I was keen to return and, regardless of my own petty feelings, I had a family to support. Naturally, nothing at work had changed when I got back, but Bernice treated me with kid gloves at the Mercy and Terri kept a close eye on me in CUH.

Most of the rest of 2011 was spent battling in the two departments and, for recreation, I engaged in feisty exchanges in the medical and general press with doctors-in-training and a consultant or two over my suggestions for getting Irish graduates to work at the frontline. My popularity with my colleagues remained low, as I continued to restate what I thought was obvious and wrong. And frankly, despite the counselling and a failed trial of antidepressant medication, my burnout and my self-inflicted woes were driving me to drink.

That was a shame, because I've never been able to drink. Initially, as a teenager, I found alcohol helped my social anxiety, the one that seems to affect so many Irish people, especially those who, like me, are deeply ashamed of their birth circumstances, home, uncertain identity and a myriad other issues. That's how I explained my intake as a youngster, anyhow, even when the drinking itself was the source of embarrassment. And then came middle age and, like many older medics, I hadn't calibrated the intake downwards as much as the science and sense would recommend. So I would tend to fall asleep at dinner parties after about three glasses of wine, which would unfortunately shift the awkwardness to my poor wife.

Still, life at home was a lot more positive than at work. Victoria was networking and helping to raise considerable funds for the city's homeless, with the Cork Simon Ball committee, and the children were thriving, especially Ciara, who'd headed off to study medicine in Galway. And my 92-year-old mother was thoroughly enjoying her relocation to Cork. She was making many new friends around her cosy new apartment in Ballinlough, and often said that she should have moved south years before. She even talked briefly about my father one afternoon over her favourite tipple, a glass of stout, in Longboats in Ballintemple, and in a matter-of-fact way confessed that her heart had been completely broken when Leslie died in 1963. I believed her, and I began to comprehend some of her stance towards my endless questions when I was younger. The truth was, she'd been grieving desperately for years.

So, what did I learn from those years in the wilderness and my battle with burnout?

Probably the greatest effect that my few psychotherapy-cum-counselling sessions had on me after the radio debacle was to encourage me to use 'I' rather than 'one' or 'we', which were always my preferred pronouns, not least because my old-fashioned mother was forever uttering the phrase, 'Self-praise is no praise'. So I'm torn, still, as I repeatedly refer to myself, hopefully with the minimum of bombast. But this book has primarily been about 'I', as well as the 'we', without whom life would not have been worth living, and it has been an exercise in honest emotional expression after years of pretending to be strong, resilient and unimpeachable.

So here goes. I was very wrong. I was wrong to keep on keeping on. I was wrong to allow my perfectionism to harm the lives of those I loved. I was really wrong to live the way I did for as long as I did. And I'm ashamed of the hurt I caused to people close to me as I abreacted to my own difficulties.

What I have learned from a brief acquaintance with the work of psychotherapists like Frank Tallis is that the legacy of 1960s' individualism − 'reaching for the stars', 'don't let anyone stop you', and 'never give up' − was a *huge ego trap*, into which I fell, headfirst, in my relentless pursuit of high-minded *perfection*. The second lesson I learned is that the pursuit of perceived success (money, celebrity, titles or even, in my case, just being 'right') is disastrously unrealistic in evolutionary terms. In short, biology requires us to belong to a community, to be hugged regularly, physically and figuratively, and to be *realistic* in our dealings with a difficult world, not endlessly tilting at windmills. The third crucial lesson I learned is that we, meaning *I*, need to create *a coherent narrative*, or a life story that makes some kind of sense to us, in order to achieve a degree of mental well-being, and what Osler called 'equanimity'.

But the overwhelming problem for me was that the story of my career as a frontline physician seemed to me ultimately to be about a messy failure. From a shameful start to a humiliating finish. Clinically, I might as well have been sending despatches from the Somme. Not quite 'nothing to see here', but who really cared about the muddied chaos of the emergency department frontline moving a few figurative feet backwards and forwards over years? And the most infuriating problems, day-in, day-out, were the perennial shortages of stock, staff and space, not exciting discoveries, miracle cures, or fantastic tales of redemption, victory or romance.

Towards the end, the more I spent time with my dear old mother, the more I learned from her late-onset serenity and equanimity, and the more I really admired her. Even at 90-odd, she cheerfully and magnificently embodied the old idea: 'When you're going through hell, keep going'. She had certainly done so, and perhaps the centre *could* hold for me too.

Overthinking It

My favourite description of adult life is the one set out on an amusing card I bought years ago in Liverpool. It goes: 'Being an adult is pretty easy. You just feel tired all the time and tell people about how tired you are, and they tell you how tired they are'. In many respects, that defined life in my mid-fifties, but I did seem to enter a spiral of physical as well as mental decline in 2012, with a steady stream of ailments. In fact, Bernice at the Mercy did seem to anticipate the issue when she said to me on my fiftieth birthday: 'You do realise, Chris, that once you hit your fifties, the wheels start to fall off?!'

The most mysterious ailment was the barking cough and breathlessness that affected me in the first half of 2012, and which progressed alarmingly after I got to Greece on holiday with the family. It got to the point where I was quite fearful of the twilight because every night, after dinner, I found myself prostrated on the villa's bathroom floor, gasping and choking between terrifying paroxysms of coughing. I've been frightened for my life a few times, like when I was addled in

Amsterdam or battling a riptide on a Queensland beach, but this suffocating cough was the most terrifying experience I'd ever had. And intriguing, too, because none of the specialist colleagues I consulted on corridors afterwards recognised the underlying disease from my description. That is, until my old mother remarked that my periodic barking sounded 'very like whooping cough'. And, lo and behold, the serology confirmed that I did indeed have the '100-day cough', or pertussis, along with thousands of others that year in Ireland, the UK and North America. I was painfully reminded that immunity after vaccination or previous infection with childhood diseases wears off. And I wasn't being melodramatic – there were two deaths that year in Ireland from the disease.

Then, in 2015, breathlessness and vague chest pains began to affect me after rugby coaching sessions on Saturdays and even modest cycling trips to Cobh. Eventually my wife dragged me to the cardiology service at the Mater Hospital, in Cork, where an angiogram was arranged. To everyone's shock, it showed a potentially lethal narrowing of one of my main coronary arteries. The sort that used to create a lot of widows. Thankfully, I was soon on the receiving end of 'the magic of medicine': a couple of stents sorted the blockage, and I was able to return to do battle at work, as well as my Sunday morning cycling trips, which were an essential balm for my burned-out brain.

Physically, then, I was better in terms of the chest pain and breathlessness, but the 'writer's cramp', a euphemism for the generalised aching and weakness of my whole right arm that came on when I wrote, was becoming quite disabling, and this was the main reason I agreed to try spinal surgery at the end of 2017, to ease the pressure on my nerves. Alas, the pain recurred some months later and I found that writing quickly or for more than about ten minutes invariably triggered the cramping, numbness and weakness. So I was in a pretty pickle, given that a core part of an emergency physician's work is seeing patients at speed, and writing accompanying notes at pace. Worse still, I wasn't able to pop the frailest elderly lady's dislocated shoulder back in. And handshakes were becoming a no-no.

So, why didn't I just call it a day? I suppose I muddled along for a bit longer because the work was so important, the clinical issues were still interesting and compelling, and I still enjoyed being part of the world of the ED. There were always new developments in toxicology for instance, like the ever-more exotic drugs being sold online or on the streets and killing people. The most tragic example of this in 2012 was the deaths of two young men in Kinsale, who'd consumed lethal amounts of MDMA and PMMA, one of the many dangerous new chemicals on the streets of our towns. Afterwards, the coroner remarked wistfully that he'd been dealing with similar deaths in Kinsale for the previous sixteen years, and he hoped lessons would be learned. But such deaths continued to multiply year after year, and some people *never* learn.

Another sort of 'progress' was in the new kind of criminal violence that exploded into the ED from time to time – the odd bloodbath in Resus after migrant gangs tried to butcher each other in Cork. In short, the stuff I'd seen in Liverpool twenty years earlier, but now being seen in every town in Ireland. I'm talking of the sort of war-zone situation I was called in for in Resus one night when I found myself leading a team of mostly young nurses in a multiple trauma scenario, who responded with exemplary efficiency to the arrival of several victims of hideous machete wounds, to the limbs, head and torso. What I found encouraging and discouraging in equal measure that evening was how thrilled the staff nurses were to be dealing with cases of real 'war medicine', rather than endlessly negotiating trolleys on a packed corridor. I could readily understand their enthusiasm, but I admit I was as fascinated by the variety of 'thug life' tattoos and pictures of Kalashnikovs on gang members' arms as I was by their gaping lacerations. I'd seen enough of those to last me a lifetime.

Thankfully, I was still buoyed up by the continuing evolution of basic emergency care, despite the difficulties. Like the use of telemedicine, for example, reviewing people at home far from the Mercy or CUH, by phone or email, rather than dragging them into congested waiting rooms. I experimented with scheduling care for people in West Cork who'd sustained minor injuries, to avoid them rushing unnecessarily to the hospital on a weekend or at night.

And I glimpsed an even more exciting future when I conducted my remotest ever teleconsultation, with the mother of a young man in the Maldives who'd been stung by a stingray. (The main thing is not to panic, and to apply heat to the sting area for up to 90 minutes!)

Increasingly, my greatest clinical enthusiasm was for the achievements of other staff, like the Interns in both EDs in Cork, and the Advanced Nurse Practitioners at CUH and the Mercy, including my brilliant 'work wife', Anne O'Keeffe, with whom I'd worked closely for many years. Truly, the handful of ANPs in Cork were delivering dramatic improvements in ambulatory care, and I came to believe that they offered Irish people a bright future of efficient, compassionate and carefully monitored care. And I said so in an enthusiastic talk to their annual conference in Dún Laoghaire in 2014. In that sense, I was vicariously enjoying the progress made in many Irish EDs by the ANPs and Interns, a situation to which I had aspired for years.

But otherwise, I fear, I was getting most of my kicks elsewhere. On the pitch at Cork Con, for instance, on Saturdays, and on the very memorable 2014 Paris Rugby Tour, for which I was the honorary medical officer, discovering for myself the hazards to the eyes and knees of the recycled rubber tyres the French use for their pitches. And the many ailments to which 13-year-old boys are prone on or off the pitch. And the delightful way in which they bounce back after injury.

One small kick was getting my prescription for a 'reboot' of EDs published in the *Irish Times* in 2015, together with an encouraging mention in the accompanying editorial. And I had another piece of good fortune when, in late 2012, I was invited to be the doctor on the new RTÉ *Today* programme, with Dáithí Ó Sé and Maura Derrane. That really was a *lot* of fun, with a great bunch of people in the studio team, and I thoroughly enjoyed demonstrating simple first-aid techniques as well as chatting about the issues of the day. It was nice, too, to be recorded on video for posterity and educational purposes on the IAEM and RTÉ websites, even if such videos are now absolutely routine in education. I remain a firm believer that medics have much to offer the population with infotainment on the radio and TV. There is, after all, so much to know, and so many ways in which a well-educated public can help the health system.

I was still enjoying the lecture circuit, too, giving talks at parent-teacher meetings in schools around Munster and

Leinster, as well as at conferences, like the huge international meeting held by the IAEM at the Dublin Conference Centre in 2012. That was a true coming-of-age event for Irish emergency medicine, with hundreds of delegates from all over the world, and a visit by our own President Michael D. Higgins.

In 2012, I attended the 30th anniversary meeting of the UCD Class of 1982, in Earslfort Terrace. It was great to meet up with old classmates who'd returned from all corners of the world, from Canada to Carlow, to sit on their 'usual' stool in Hartigan's, in Leeson Street, some of them for the first time in years. I was especially delighted to bump into old friends who had found new human or recreational passions in their later lives, often moving into intriguingly different post-medical careers. This seemed particularly vital later, at the anniversary banquet, when pictures of the numerous members of our class who'd died since graduation were projected onto the ballroom wall. That was a sobering moment, and one that concentrated many minds.

In the midst of a failing career, even one with a few extracurricular highlights, I confess that death became another important teacher. Not 'intimations of my own mortality' as such, but the accumulating deaths of people who mattered to me. People in my UCD class, like the hugely popular Mick O'Connor, who died accidentally in Liverpool, and many others named at our reunion. Close medical friends in Liverpool, Edward Kadzombe and Paul Mullins, also tragically young. Friends who were consultants in emergency medicine of a similar age to me, like Conor Egleston and Patrick Hyland-Maguire. Friends from my Dalkey days, like Johnny Piggott, Kieran Sheehan and Terry Quinn, and from school days, like John Larchet, Alan Mathews and

Hugh Howard. And, of course, the deaths in my parents' generation, like my beloved Oonagh Hayes, Bernard Share, Billy Bolger, and my own mentor, Niall O'Donohoe, who I'd visited just a day or two before he died and whose obituary I was truly honoured to write.

I always used to laugh whenever Dáithí Ó Sé mockingly addressed me as 'Monsignor' in the Cork RTÉ studio, as if I were a paragon of virtue simply because I was giving a little idealistic medical advice on the *Today* programme. But the truth is that my USP for years at work, and in debate, was that I was 'a sinner serving other sinners'. In fact, my talks to parents were popular precisely because I advertised myself as a superannuated party animal, not a finger-wagging moraliser, and self-deprecating humour was my schtick. But another truth was that, at home, I was becoming a pity-party animal, crushed by my unpopularity, burnout and the endless pain in my neck and arm, and I was self-medicating with booze. I wasn't smoking weed, I wasn't snorting lines, and I wasn't chasing women, but I was spending more and more of my off-duty time slumped on the sofa, nursing a glass of claret. And I was wracked with terrible disappointment at my disintegrating career. Worst of all, I was subjecting my family to increasingly frequent, thoughtless and unjustifiable angry outbursts.

Then, in 2014, I had the luckiest break of all. Watching a recording of the *Today* programme, I finally 'saw' myself on TV and thought: *That guy really is pity-partying much too hard for a man of his age, he looks exhausted, flushed and overweight.*

And, because I was genuinely 'blessed among women', because I had an unreasonably loyal and loving wife, mother, daughters, secretaries and a first-class GP to support me, I actually learned the obvious lesson, the need for a radical change in lifestyle, and that year I started to turn the tanker around. I also had the support of my *consigliere*, David, and the rest of the lads when I announced to them all that I had given up both drinking and moaning. What was wonderful was that they were all so enthusiastic about the new, happier me. And it was hugely encouraging, on each annual Camino trip, to be told that I always seemed to be in great form. And, after a while, it became a doddle. I was much less angry, I slept better, I felt better, and I *was* better.

It also became much easier to be more realistic about work. I began to ease up on myself, and my unreasonable expectations. I stopped worrying that managers and colleagues were avoiding me. The conditions were atrocious, but I accepted that I could only do so much, particularly as I continued to struggle with my neck and dodgy arm. And if staff came and went, I saw it as an understandable, even necessary reality that people would do as much as they could in our EDs and move on when they'd done what they could. I began to spot how many other friends and colleagues had subtly adjusted their work-life balance after years at the frontline, too. Some moved sideways, into management, committee or college work, or became academics, all of which meant fewer patient contacts. Sadly, the truth is that corrosion in emergency healthcare is correlated with the number of patient contacts. Other friends even left the speciality, to embark on different medical and non-medical careers.

And, as for me, I finally resolved to write this book – a sort of apology for and explanation of 'where it all went wrong' – in 2019, as I lay squirming on a pain specialist's table, slowly inhaling the familiar antiseptic fumes, ignoring the ominous tearing of packaging and silently intoning of a phrase I'd heard so often in the Dublin of my youth: 'Me nerves have me ruined.' The good doctor was stabbing me again and again in the neck with a long, fine needle as he probed for a precise spot around my spine in which to inject his anaesthetic cocktail. The poking was startlingly sore and in between wincing and gritting my teeth, I was also reflecting on that little slogan that I'd recited endlessly in my emergency departments for years, to anyone who'd listen: *Happiness is the absence of pain.* I found myself thinking that this idea should really (ouch, again!) be conveyed to every single medical student and nurse.

And yet the procedure itself wasn't the cause of my mounting distress, so much as the dawning realisation that, not only was my dear old mother about to die in the coming hours, but my right hand was now paralysed. Not entirely, in fairness, but I didn't think I could raise my wrist off the trolley where it rested without having to vigorously shrug my shoulder or neck. Sudden movement would have been disastrous, however, as the tip of the needle was disconcertingly close to my spinal cord. Nor was it just the weakness of my hand that perturbed me. It was the thought that I desperately needed to get back to the unfolding death-bed scene in the nursing home, not far from where her only offspring was already laid out, under green surgical drapes. And then – with the same hand – draft some sort of outline of the service, eulogy and sacred melodies with which I hoped to send my dying parent back to her Maker, in the coming days.

In my defence, I didn't proceed beyond polite mumbled protest to full panic mode. At my advanced stage in life, I'd experienced enough painful procedures, and crises, to realise that this needling, too, would pass. And yet the prospect of being unable to type, or write, while trying to organise a funeral, and all that that entailed, was a cause of rapidly mounting, strangely childish dismay. In truth, I wasn't making my calculations at that point as an emergency physician, who had himself punctured countless patients with needles and knives, but as a suddenly, intensely anxious, middle-aged only child, finally about to be orphaned.

'Eh, Tony?', I muttered to my brilliant and carefully chosen colleague.

'Yes?'

'You know I've no movement in my right hand?'

There was silence, as my comrade looked at me quizzically over his face mask, seemingly momentarily uncertain if I was actually medically qualified.

'Ah, Chris, you're overthinking it!', he chortled, as he withdrew the needle for the last time, gently removed the surgical drapes and pronounced the procedure to be at an end.

Finally, I was able to shrug my shoulder, and confirm with my own eyes that I was indeed in possession of a florid 'wrist drop', or paralysis. But, more importantly, the pain above my shoulder blade had dwindled to a mere ache, and there was the prospect of escape. Happiness, indeed. In fact, more than that. Bliss.

The relief afterwards in the recovery area was intense, as the power in my upper limb slowly returned, and the cheery nursing staff fussed over me with tea and TLC. My normally reliable black humour resurfaced, too, as I reflected that, like politicians, pain specialists really *don't get your pain*. And, of course, they mustn't – because surgeons have to be the sort who are happy to stick the knife in, emergency physicians need to be crazy stress junkies with short attention spans, and so on. Because when you do think about it, as I then did, that's the way it's got to be if medics are to do their job.

And as I've long realised, having dealt with so many people in crisis, most of us don't even try to put ourselves in others' shoes. There are too many shoes. And too little time. So why would Tony have been focusing on anything other than the anatomy of my neck, where the spinal nerve roots emerge to enable precise movement and sensation in the upper limbs? Or sometimes, not quite enable, as in my case, where these 'wires' had been damaged as they squeezed through ever-narrower gaps between discs and bone. Why? The mundane answer is wear and tear, or degenerative cervical spondylosis, to be precise, which is of course due to *Anno Domini* (i.e. advancing old age), as I've explained to many patients with the same problem. Plus, decades of having shoulder and neck muscles stretched as taut as violin strings in the permanent war zone that is your average hospital emergency department.

So Tony was right. I *was* overthinking it. As per usual. Even though I should have been well aware that injecting anaesthetic around the nerves causing my intermittent but disabling arm pain might alleviate the discomfort, the cost would be a negative impact on the adjacent nerves that supply power to the same limb. And, as the weakness predictably resolved, I realised with embarrassment that my alarm was misplaced, irrational and bizarrely naïve.

But, as I said before, I live in fear. Always have done, in retrospect. Which may seem a barely credible thing for a frontline physician to claim, especially one who has spent so much time contending with routinely challenging, sometimes terrifying, situations. And I have myself undertaken treatments that seemed a little brutal, or nerve-racking, at the time, to me and the patient. However, the endless purposeful activity of a busy doctor is at least a partial remedy for their own fear, anxiety or insecurity. A carefully honed empathy, a ceaseless concern for others, can mean less self-obsession, less time to dwell on doubt, or rumination as psychiatrists call it. This very ability to do something beneficial for others was probably what allowed, or even compelled, me to endure so many years in medical trench warfare. By which I mean those infernally overcrowded Irish, English and Scottish hospital emergency departments where I worked for years, with steadily worsening shortages of staff, space and time. Not to mention the ever-growing intensity, complexity and volume of crises, in deplorable conditions, and a fug of fear and loathing that so often engulfed staff and patients.

And then, as my wife collected me an hour or so after my spinal injections, a fully-fledged, authentically vulnerable patient, I faced the greatest fear of all. The death of my mother. Finally, after years of dreading precisely this moment, it had arrived. And still I wasn't sure if I was ready. Maybe I'd crack up. Who knew? Or maybe, as my comrade had put it, I was simply – as always – overthinking it, overfeeling it, and overreacting to it.

As it turned out, I managed to get back to St Luke's Home, by Cork's great tree-rimmed estuary, an hour or so later and, as my wrist weakness resolved over a few hours, I got to hold the hand of my remarkable mother, Colette Redmond, as her life ebbed away. Made of the finest Dublin steel, she lasted a further 40 hours, and her peaceful death was that wonderful thing – a blessed release after years of frailty, falls and total blindness. And, although she died at the grand old age of 99 without ever managing to say 'I love you' to me, I didn't crack up. Because by then, I was finally convinced that she did. She had rescued me, supported me, endorsed me for the duration of my sentient existence and, in the end, I realised that her actions – those of a genuine lioness – had long since provided *proof* of a love that was beyond any amount of sentimental words. Show, don't tell, they say.

In my heartfelt, and momentarily tearful, eulogy in St Joseph's Church in Ballintemple a few days after she died, I proclaimed to friends, family and former hospital colleagues that what modest success I might have had in my life, and in my 35 years in emergency medicine, I owed to my mother. And quite a bit of the irrational fear, too, to be fair.

And so it was at the end of my 'first career' as a medic that, after a certain amount of death, decay and disintegration caught up with me, I had time to learn from my experience. And with the help of a patient counsellor, an exceptionally compassionate GP, and a loving partner, I arrived at a point where I finally accepted I'd done as much as I could. The occupational health assessment was that I was so disabled by my neck decay and resulting nerve damage that I couldn't perform all the duties required of an emergency physician. I did explore the possibility of working in another area of the health service, but that wasn't on offer and, while I felt it was a sad waste of my experience, I agreed to take early retirement in 2018, not far off my sixtieth birthday. It was a far cry from the glory I'd dreamed of in my youth, but I had struggled on for as long as I could. And I'd done the best that I could.

For a long time, I felt ashamed of my failure as a doctor. If the truth be known, I experienced the sort of shame that had haunted and humiliated me as a boy and teenager. But then I remembered that, unlike so many people I'd loved and admired, I was still alive. Unlike so many people, I'd been exceptionally lucky to have had my heart and head problems spotted and sorted. And unlike some middle-aged men in crisis, feeling lost and alone, I was surrounded by a wonderful family, who were determined to support me in my new existence, who coaxed me out of the slough of despond, and who were delighted that I had 'retired', so long as I wasn't at home during office hours.

Even so, it has taken me a long while to recover from leaving the trenches, where I had been so determined for so long to lead from the front, honourably and – above all – dependably. The disappointment at not being able to continue doing my duty was the hardest part of leaving, as was not being around so many admirable and congenial comrades. Ironically, the most gratifying few words of validation came from my friend, former colleague, and the country's Chief Clinical Officer, Dr Colm Henry, who described me, in a farewell Tweet in 2018, as 'Thinker, Innovator, Contrarian'. I could really have done with those words when the sky fell in on my head in 2011, but better late than never!

And I'm glad to say that in 2021 the burnout has largely been resolved. Just as the Medical Protection Society anticipated, getting away from my chaotic and challenging workplaces was the primary treatment I required. And I'm equally pleased to say that I am not suffering from Post-Traumatic Stress Disorder, a different but just as onerous a burden for so many who work in emergency departments. Indeed, while the issue of burnout needs to be considered very carefully and very urgently if the staffing shortages in the acute health service are to be remedied, the 'vicious circle' of *emotional trauma – career trauma – emotional trauma* at the frontline also needs to be recognised. I am convinced that many people choose a career at the 'pointy end' of healthcare because of their own - sometimes traumatic - back story: but this should not be mistaken as a need for *more* trauma. Quite the opposite. I think there is a desire among such staff to prevent trauma to others, and simply to care for those suffering from trauma and other sources of severe pain and distress.

I have learned many hard lessons from a life at the healthcare frontline way, and another important one was that, even if there were a few people who caused difficulty for me, such individuals exist in every walk of life, and such friction comes with being a member of the species of *Homo sapiens*. And even if angry exchanges are a shockingly common feature of hospital life everywhere, I have long come to understand that most people are only aggressive when they're feeling fearful or overwhelmed. Moreover, as the old saying goes, resentment is like taking poison and waiting for the object of your bitterness to fall sick. So, I recognise that *I* was the primary author of most of the 'misfortune' I experienced during what was otherwise a wonderful few decades, caring for other members of my species. I now understand that most of it was due to that 'overthinking, overfeeling and overreacting', which is just what I do.

However, by far the most painful lesson I have learned from the past 40 medical years was that my mental, physical and emotional exhaustion was desperately hard on those closest to me, who saw me morph into a black-and-white negative of my former self, distracted, uncommunicative and buried in despair. And the greatest pleasure I now get in life is in renewing, refreshing and nurturing old and new relationships. I believe indeed that these are ultimately the source of the greatest happiness in any human's life. All I have to do now is to live for another 30 years, reinvent myself, and who knows what I might achieve.

Carpe diem? Definitely.

Epilogue: Hope Springs

Eighteen months after my retirement from clinical work, as the world witnessed the relentless spread of the worst pandemic in a century, people in Ireland watched in horror as truckloads of elderly dead were transported nightly from well-resourced but overwhelmed hospitals in Lombardy, and the Irish health service was placed on the highest level of alert to deal with the predicted devastation here. In an unrehearsed radio interview in March 2020, when the presenter asked me if I would answer 'Ireland's call' to recently retired doctors to return to the healthcare frontline, I said I'd do so gladly. Just a few days later, I received a phone call from Dr Kieran O'Connor, Clinical Director of the Mercy Hospital, asking if I'd consider returning to work in the ED. I agreed immediately.

It was hugely gratifying to be as warmly received back in the Mercy as I was, not least of all by my former colleague, now lead consultant in emergency medicine in Cork, Professor Conor Deasy, who phoned me on my first day back.

'Hi, Chris! Welcome home!' he exclaimed.

'Thanks, Conor. What about you? Are you shattered?' I asked, referring to the superhuman efforts I knew he'd been making in the city's other emergency department, at CUH, ready for the anticipated onslaught of COVID-19 cases.

'Shattered? No! But I'm really excited,' he replied, enthusiastically.

'You know what?' I said. 'You're sick. But guess what, I'm excited too!'

And I truly *was* exhilarated. And delighted, too, to be of some use again. And what was even better was that the ED was initially relatively quiet, as people anxiously avoided hospitals while the numbers of coronavirus cases soared.

For me, the most remarkable thing was that I felt none of the anger that had gripped me for most of the last few years in the same hospital (and at CUH) as I'd battled with an unmanageable workload, speed-dating patients in insane conditions, while I crumbled, physically and mentally, and friends and colleagues my age and younger were dying. And I felt no fear. It was as if I'd been briefly restored to my excitable and excited twenties and thirties, with the insatiable appetite for work I'd once had, along with limitless energy and a capacity for extracting pleasure and satisfaction from every single case that presented to the ED.

It occurred to me that, in the eighteen months since I'd taken early retirement, after 35 years at the pointy end of healthcare, I'd accommodated the two events I had most dreaded: my mother's death, and the premature demise of a once-promising career. And then, still overthinking it, I reflected on the childhood origins of my intense lifelong anxiety, and its relationship with a career in a hyper-stressful sphere of healthcare, i.e. emergency medicine, the scary, chaotic, vital medical care that goes on in hospitals, refugee camps, city streets and battlefields, real and notional, around the world.

I thought of all the wonderful professionals with whom I'd worked over the years, and I recalled how so many of them had also been forced out too soon from careers at the same sharp end of healthcare. And how most of them must have gone through similar stages of exhilaration, exasperation, exhaustion and crippling demotivation in the course of their years in an emergency department, or related service. It struck me that the very best of them were no less anxious than me, in the staffroom or hospital car park, and no less grimly determined approaching the Resus Room or accident scene. Most importantly, I was reminded that *people are not logical, they are biological.* So, like me on the specialist's couch, what sometimes drove them was the subconscious after-effects of an adverse childhood or early adult experience. And I was left thinking that this is an extraordinarily important - unforgettable - consideration in recruiting people to our health service, because the very thing that motivates them to care passionately for others is what makes them vulnerable to burnout or post-traumatic stress - if their professional burden is not carefully monitored and calibrated to their capability (including the inevitable decline with age).

In the end, my hands-on pandemic experience in 2020 was relatively short. I retired again from the frontline after a few months, once the first wave and its associated stress had abated, and I watched from a distance as the national response in Ireland waxed and waned, stumbled, shot ahead of other countries, and then fell back again. And, just as I had anticipated at the outset, it turned out to be *truly* historic.

Just like the First World War, it wasn't 'over by Christmas', as was first predicted. And it did resemble a composite of the Spanish Flu of 1918–1919 and the first pandemic of the 21st century, SARS, insofar as it crept up on countries all over the world, and the ones that were best prepared were the countries that had recently experienced the medical and financial impact of SARS in 2003, like South Korea and Hong Kong. There, surveillance teams, testing and quarantining set up after SARS were rapidly deployed. So, as I write, the world continues to battle with COVID-19, with endless international squabbling over vaccine production, funding and logistics, and the disease is likely to come and go in waves for a few more years, until global herd immunity is genuinely achieved.

However, even in the midst of an exhausting pandemic, with all its privations and miseries, I am frequently reminded that the word *apocalypse* derives from the Greek for *revelation*. So, for months now, I've been struck by the enormous number of discoveries, or re-discoveries, that have been going on since February 2020.

Lest we forget, that was when the pandemic displaced the seismic reverberations of Ireland's general election from our airwaves and Letters pages. And I am very hopeful that some of these re/discoveries may help transform the post-apocalyptic world for the better. They include the surge in urban growing of vegetables, micro-gardens on apartment block balconies ('plots in the sky'), as well as along canals and on carpark rooftops. Already, the reports of 'horticultural healing', in these oases amid the concrete, are really encouraging, and I note that doctors are increasingly prescribing gardening for its proven benefits in combating anxiety, depression and loneliness – one of the major public health threats of the post-modern world – not to mention food security and climate change.

I am also hugely optimistic about the potential for Zoom, or similar video-conferencing platforms, in future healthcare. When I look back at the number of hours I've spent walking over to HR offices to do interviews, driving to another hospital in the city to give early morning tutorials to a few latecomers, or taking the train to Dublin for just one meeting, and I consider how many stressful, time-consuming, CO_2-emitting journeys might have been avoided with this technology, I'm genuinely excited. Such teleconferencing could save thousands of hours of medical and administrative time, and hundreds of tonnes of CO_2 emissions, in Ireland alone.

And that's only the half of it. For years, I've jested that surgery used to be called 'trauma by appointment', and I argued that there was no good reason why many people couldn't have an *appointment for their trauma* (or minor injuries) with the right amount of organisation. My own version of this was enabling GPs or other colleagues to make an appointment in my Rapid Access Clinic for certain patients (with fresh or complicated injuries) to see me directly, rather than spend half a weekend in a cramped waiting room to see a sometimes-inexperienced doctor. This approach worked well, but the problem was that for a long time there was only me to provide the service. Then the Advanced Nurse Practitioners in the Mercy ED began to schedule appointments informally, and the results have been really promising. It means that people don't always have to spend hours in a waiting room, but can see an expert in injury care at a mutually suitable time. I think the next stage of evolution will be the review of patients by video-conferencing. This will allow a little forward-planning to creep into ED care, and a great deal of review or follow-up might be done this way, from the patient's home or perhaps a GP Practice Nurse's office. In any event, the potential for transforming emergency care is vast. Already, American medics are saying that 'telemedicine is the new house call'.

A third revelation of the pandemic has been the extraordinary collaboration and healthy rivalry between scientists and laboratories all over the world in producing vaccines against the coronavirus. Creating old-style vaccines with bits of virus usually takes years, so to have created vaccines within months is remarkable, albeit with massive government support. And then there are the 'messenger' and 'self-amplifying RNA' vaccines, which are a whole new approach that may allow relatively easy tweaking to deal with new variants of the coronavirus, *and* other major diseases. The future for vaccinology is intensely bright and, hopefully, similar global scientific cooperation can continue in future, in new TB, malaria and cancer treatments, and indirectly in slowing climate change.

In truth, then, I'm pretty upbeat about the acute health sector in the coming years. I've been up close to the inner workings of the HSE in recent months, and I'm genuinely encouraged by observing the talented people rising to the top in the health service. Moreover, I think the population-wide approach to resource use during the pandemic has provided a vital shake-up of strategic thinking. It has obliged politicians and the populace to accept the *limitations* of our capabilities, and to appreciate that evidence-based *priorities* are vital to medical effectiveness *and* a sense of fairness. For instance, in the present pandemic, we now know that age is the paramount risk factor that trumps all others by a long way. And the devastating cyberattack on the country's health system in May 2021 has surely left no one in any doubt about the fragility of our systems. There may be gripes about elderly software, but it was interesting to see how few people blamed 'the government' on this occasion. There can have been fewer more painful lessons of late around the harsh reality of our hyperconnected and globalised world, which is not just about the convenience of 'click and collect' but also one which leaves us all at the mercy of cybercriminals and other terrifyingly powerful hostile actors. I truly hope that – after the spectacular combination of pandemic and cyberattack – people will be a little more understanding of the challenges of healthcare in the 21st century. I certainly get that 'vibe' when I meet more and more people who have been efficiently vaccinated in recent months, and who are extremely grateful to the system, and the way it has 'upped its game'.

I am even more optimistic, in fact I'm very excited, about the future of emergency medicine in Ireland. I believe we are actually on the cusp of a golden age for the specialty. This may sound a little odd coming from a casualty of burnout, who has been complaining about conditions in the country's EDs for years *and* battling to fix them. But timing really is everything. My timing wasn't ideal, because it takes time to develop a discipline and a brand, in just the same way as it takes time to plan, fund and commission new buildings.

Forty years ago, emergency medicine was an emerging discipline, populated by distinctly unusual types of doctor, including those with a background in military and missionary medicine, who were attracted to the chaos at the door of most hospitals. When I stepped onto the stage, the regular troupe of emergency physicians was probably enough to mount a two-hander in the back of the local pub. Now, a highly disciplined and proud regiment of emergency medics could put on a huge show in the National Concert Hall, with an enormous cast, to a full house. Better still, there is a growing queue of enthusiastic medical students getting into the emergency medicine groove even before they qualify. And what the specialty has achieved in the past few decades is remarkable.

Not only has it seen a transformation in the care of heart attacks, strokes, diabetic and respiratory crises, meningitis, septicaemia and, of course, trauma in all its guises, but it has driven extraordinary progress in pre-hospital care, where Ireland is now beginning to compete with long-established systems in Europe, North America and Australia. It is truly amazing to see the sort of intensive care that Jason Van Der Velde, Adrian Murphy and Hugh Doran deliver at the side of the road throughout Cork county. Similar work is happening in Wicklow, Donegal and other parts of the country. And, in 2021, other types of care in the community are provided by ED doctors going out to the homes of elderly people in Cork and Dublin, assessing their needs after an emergency call, and keeping many of them out of busy EDs.

The organisation of emergency medicine nationally has also made giant leaps forward: the IAEM is now capable of running spectacular international and national conferences and relentlessly promotes public debate on overcrowding and public health matters. And the progress in academic and research terms has been equally impressive, with Professors of Emergency Medicine now to be found in most teaching hospitals, many of them running major research projects, as well as the National Office for Clinical Audit (the prime provider of evidence for health policymakers). And I can safely say that the splendid regiment of future and present emergency physicians in this country is already deploying the energy, experience and vision required to place it in the top ranks of emergency care in the near future. And that is a wonderful thing to be able to say.

For my own part, I would encourage future medical students and graduates to think about a career in emergency medicine. It is an incredibly exciting specialty and there really is little to beat the sense of real achievement, the easing of human suffering and 'doing the right thing' that is so readily available at the frontline. And before people say, *But what about what happened to you?*, I must acknowledge that I had my own personal difficulties *long* before I made my career choice. And I again admit freely that I was the author of most of my own misfortunes. I clearly suffered from the dysfunctional perfectionism that is at the root of so much dissatisfaction in the medical profession. And timing *is* everything. My single greatest mistake, the one that caused me most difficulty, was simply signing a killer-contract that obliged me to work in three separate hospitals at once. This was like playing part-time for three rival football teams and agreeing to build a new clubhouse at each ground. Many people warned me it would be disastrous and, in fact, around 2006 the whole idea of multi-site working for consultants was described as unsustainable. Sadly, I was living proof of that.

In my defence, in 1999, the move back to Ireland seemed to be the one and only way I could get back on the island after nearly fourteen years in exile. And, in the end, while it was a professionally retrograde move, one could argue that all careers eventually end in failure. And the dubious career move actually meant that I got to share the last two decades of my mother's life with her. There were many challenges, of course, like her blindness and frailty, but I'm certain that she had an incomparably happier last twenty years than she would have had if I'd stayed overseas to pursue professional glory. Not only that, but we got to spend many happy hours together, as she reminisced and I listened, and I finally succeeded in devising a 'coherent narrative' for her, too.

In hindsight, my mother had had a very unhappy childhood with her own difficult mother (who herself started life in the tenements in Dublin) but, by the late 1950s, she'd found a job for life and the love of her life. And even though she could never have had him all to herself, it became clear to me that she was determined to arrive at some sort of compromise. And then, in quick succession, she (temporarily) lost her baby boy, she lost the love of her life and she lost the job she loved and at which she excelled. Life dealt her a cruel hand of cards and, unsurprisingly, she suffered from terrible grief in the 1960s and 1970s. But she just got on with it. My mother was herself sometimes described as 'difficult', because she could be acerbic in her comments, but I still think that in different circumstances she could have been President of Ireland, given her remarkable brain power, ability and shining decency. And the more I got to know her, the more I understood the critical role of difficulty in *her* life. I am proud to say that, in sharing her final years with her family, and watching her grandchildren grow into fine young people, she achieved a sort of serenity or, dare I say it, a happy *equanimity*, for which I am eternally grateful. It is not everybody, after all, who gets to 'fix' many of the difficulties of their childhood, the way my mother and I did in the end.

Among her many legacies, real and metaphorical, the one that made perhaps the greatest immediate difference was what, in May 2021, I found tucked amid bills in that same old filing cabinet from my childhood that my mother left behind when she died. This was a collection of newspaper cuttings with tributes paid to my father on the week he died in 1963, which, unlike the love letters, she had not burned. And they were a wondrous discovery. For most of my life, I suspected that my mother's reluctance to talk of my father was because he was some kind of likeable rogue. Or worse. In fact, Leslie Luke turned out to have been loved by both men and (too many) women. He was highly esteemed in the world of business, PR and transport, and former colleagues described him as great company, incredibly charming, meticulous, dutiful, with 'a big round head full of bright ideas' and a boyish appetite for approval. He was also a significant innovator, having created the *Harp* magazine, co-founded the Institute of Public Relations of Ireland (now PRII) and established the first Irish News Agency, which only foundered for want of capital in an impoverished post-war Ireland. The tributes hinted at the loss of a great talent when he died suddenly, aged just 48. I have found it hard to express just how relieved I was to read all this pre-Internet material for the first time. Even belatedly, it has given me immense satisfaction to get to 'know' my father better, and to find out that – a weakness for the opposite sex aside – he was a good man, with high hopes, who was all too human.

Such things really matter, because as Oscar Wilde famously said: 'Children begin by loving their parents; after a time they judge them; rarely if ever do they forgive them'.

In February 2021, I watched the many middle-aged Irish men and women on the RTÉ *Prime Time Investigates* programme, still weeping as they recalled how they were taken from their mothers before being trafficked by adoption agencies and children's homes in the 1950s and 1960s. A few months later, I know that I was utterly blessed to have been reunited with my own mother in the 1960s, and – even belatedly – to have come to partially know, forgive, and still love two parents.

And now, in 2021, while I might feel I was prematurely wrenched from my modest career, I realise that for as long as it lasted, it was a magical and meaningful journey, working with magnificent people, all of us fighting the good fight. To paraphrase the Talking Heads, I find myself now with a beautiful wife, and four wonderful children whom I adore, and I ask, yet again, *How did I get here?* I count it unquestionably as the other great achievement of my life to have been able to show my old mother the love she deserved from her only son. After all, what is more natural than love between life partners, parents and offspring? And what is lovelier than reconciliation?

It was Freud, that archetypal investigator of childhood's legacies, who said, 'One day, in retrospect, the years of struggle will strike you as the most beautiful'. How right he was.

Acknowledgements

The first person I must thank (or should I say blame?!) for persuading me to write this book is my friend and now veteran author, Brian O'Connell, who also introduced me to the lovely Faith O'Grady at the Lisa Richards Agency, without whose belief and generous encouragement the process would never have started. I must also thank Sarah Liddy and her wonderful team at Gill, Rachel Pierce, Rachel Thompson, Laura King and Sheila Armstrong, for affording me the opportunity to publish my memoirs, as well as their saintly forbearance and firm but steady guidance throughout the exercise. And a special 'Thank you!' to my wife, Victoria, and children, Ciara, Naoise, Aoibhe and Harrison, without whose love, laughter and general lippiness I could not have survived, or thrived.

Only children are forever inventing relatives, it is said. And I immediately put my own hands up. There are a myriad individuals who – over six decades – have provided me with the sort of 'familial' love and affection which have made my life so unexpectedly worthwhile, but I must name my most cherished pseudo-relations: the Hayes family of Stillorgan Grove (especially my 'surrogate mum' Oonagh, Jarlath, Dara, Susan, Hilary, Ruth and Bronwyn), the Shares of Killiney (Jill, Bernard, Perry and Tristram), the Quinns of Glenageary (Rita, Bill, Terry and Rosaleen), the Bolgers of Donnybrook (Eithne, Billy, and Mary Ann), the Victorys of Brewery Road (Geraldine, Gerald, Alma, Fiona, Isolde, Ray and Alan), the Kennys of Dún Laoghaire (Ruth, Edmond, John, Vanessa,

Peter, Jeremy and Sarah), the Noones of Glenageary (Doreen, Paddy, Matt, David, Joe, Kathy and Paul), the O'Donohoes of Dartry (Barbara, Niall, Simon, Nick, David, Richard and Alan), the Wilkies of Edinburgh (David, Marie, Marijane, Jackie and Vicky), as well as the Vards of Sandyford, the Darraghs of Dún Laoghaire (especially David and Ed), the Clearys of Sutton, and the Ryans of Mount Merrion. I offer my thanks too to my mother's most loyal non-work friends: Grainne Marnell, Caitlin O'Byrne, Mary Dolan, Kay Conway, Sylvia Byrne, Nellie Walsh, Beatrice Reid, Gertie Redmond, and Ada Kelly.

I am also keen to identify the fraternity of friends who've kept me going – and laughing – since the 1960s, including the Oaktree Road Gang in Stillorgan: Eugene (Nudge) Harrington, John and Stephen Conway, David Delahunt, James Dormer, and – ex officio – Allan Gannon; my treasured friends and pseudo-siblings from school in the 1960s, who currently constitute the St Conleth's College Camino Club: Ray Victory, Peter Kenny, David O'Donohoe, Mark O'Donovan, Damien Neylin, Richard O'Donohoe and Julian Carvill; and former Conlethians, Alan O'Donohoe, John Larchet, Michael Ryan, Anthony Keane, Simon MacGowan, Tom de Brit, Fergal Anderson, Declan Cullen, John Nestor, Tony Cleary, David Davison, Alan Matthews, and John Carvill. I owe an incalculable debt to Michael Gardiner, Peter Gallagher and Kevin Golden for their inspiring tuition at St Conleth's. I know I was an authentically terrible 'messer', but the efforts of these Renaissance men were not in vain.

I am immeasurably grateful for a lifetime of friendship with the Glenageary ('Nurney') and Sandycove crowd from the 1970s, including John Glynn, Joe Noone, the uber-inspirational lovebirds Gordon and Lizanne Barry, Noel Casserly, Kieran Sheehan, and Carl and Carolyn Jordan. And – with the same provenance – I particularly want to thank my absurdly loyal friend, Jack Fitzgerald, of Dalkey and parts foreign, who has been a source of countless late-night laughs and good times, from Bordeaux to Ballintemple, often when I most needed them. And thanks too to Madame Alexandrine Fitzgerald for her generosity to the Lukes over the decades.

I thank my former Best Man, fellow cast member in UCD DramSoc, principal tutor in the 'Doheny and Nesbitt sessions', distinguished librarian, comic genius and genealogist, Hugh Comerford, for bearing with me during good times and bad, and for his invaluable help in tracing my ancestry. And thanks too to Sheila Miley, aka Mrs Comerford, for a friendship that goes back even further, to Ballinskelligs, circa 1974. And I thank David Valentine, my older and theoretically wiser medical classmate from UCD and the Hartigan's Annexe, former flatmate in Edinburgh, locum half-brother, and source of wit, wisdom, and the original and best 'wide-mouthed frog' story.

There were over a hundred medical students in my graduation year in UCD in 1982, but I single out a few to thank them for their affection and company, especially during my years of deep ambivalence towards medical school, as well as at the major and minor reunions of recent years: Declan Sheerin, Rosemary Rooney, Gerry Sweeney, Bryan Lynch, Garrett Igoe, Liam Farrell, Dick Hackett, Kieran McCormack, Tommy Flynn, Michael Cushen, Catherine and Robert Stuart, Stephen Cusack, Rosemary Keane, Mick Lee, Joe Duggan, John Lyons, Brian O'Connell, Fiona Donnelly, John Rice, Andy McCarthy, Justin Geoghegan,

Hugh Brady, Michael Fitzgerald, Mick Fitzpatrick, Bridin Cannon, Eithne MacMahon, Andy McCarthy, Brian Cloak, Sandra Egan, Richard Quigley, Oscar Daly, and Fergal McGoldrick.

I've had the privilege and pleasure of working with hundreds of admirable medics in Ireland, Scotland, England, and Australia, and I benefitted immensely from electives in Monaghan County Hospital and Zambia. Again, I can only accommodate a few names, but I particularly thank my inspirational (but usually unwitting) mentors: Sr Lucy O'Brien in Monze, Zambia; Mr Gordon Watson in Waterford; Professors Niall O'Higgins, Brian Maurer, and Michael Hutchison at St Vincent's Hospital in Dublin; Messrs G Angus Lee and Johnny O'Sullivan in Wexford County Hospital; Mr Frank Ward at St James' Hospital, Dublin; Mr Frank Dowling at Our Lady's Hospital for Sick Children, in Crumlin; Professor Niall V O'Donohoe of TCD, Harcourt Street and Our Lady's Hospital for Sick Children in Crumlin (my own medical guardian angel); Professor John Fennell, of St Columcille's Hospital, Loughlinstown; Dr Keith Little, Dr David Steedman, and Professor Colin Robertson of the Royal Infirmary of Edinburgh; Professor Gerry Fitzgerald of Queensland University of Technology; Professor Eamonn Quigley at UCC; and – most especially – the inimitable Dr Trevor Bayley and Dr Lawrence H Jaffey in Liverpool, who did more than any other colleagues to enable me to flourish as a young emergency physician.

I acknowledge the pleasure of working with countless other healthcare professionals in many hospitals since the start of the 1980s and I particularly thank those in Wexford, Dublin, Edinburgh, Liverpool and Cork for their friendship and support. My mother was herself a secretary and trainer of secretaries, and I want to express my particular appreciation for the secretarial assistance of a few stalwarts, including Liz MacDonald, secretary extraordinaire at the Royal Infirmary of Edinburgh; the incomparable Howard Morris, Gill, Angela, Pauline, Paula and Hazel at the Royal in Liverpool; my 'right-hand woman' at Cork University Hospital for two decades – the magnificent Terri Goulding, the indomitable Bernice O'Regan at the Mercy, and that irrepressible source of encouragement, Alethea Mansfield. I also thank Sara Mongan, Ada Hickey, Anne Fernandes and Kathleen Foley for their great patience! And thanks too to Pat Murray, Nick Ingle, Sheila Westhorp, Anita Thomas and Edna McCafferty at the Royal A&E Department for whose affection in the Nineties, I remain eternally grateful.

I have worked with and admired too many wonderful nurses to name, but I want to particularly acknowledge those who kept me going in recent years especially, including the doyenne of emergency nursing in Munster, Sheila Wall, and Mary Barry at CUH who did so much for me in 1999 and since. I thank my 'work wife' at the Mercy, Anne O'Keeffe, my 'guardian angel' at CUH, Anna Dillon, and the other Advanced Nurse Practitioners who showed me the future: Val Small, Rachel Crusher, Patrick Cotter, Ger White, Sile Stack and Sonya Healy. I thank Anne Healy for her peerless dedication, in the Mercy ED, since the beginning, Sinead Dullea for her encouragement and, also at the Mercy, my two favourite Directors of Nursing, Mary Dunnion and Margaret McKiernan. And, at the start, Eileen O'Donovan at the Mercy and Nuala Coughlan at the South Infirmary, and their crews, who were so welcoming, and such a pleasure to work with. Other nurses I should name include Alice, Ann, Anna, Anne, Annemarie, Aine, Adele, Aideen, Aisling, Amanda, Angela, Anilegna, Antoinette, Aoife, Alison, Avril, Barbara, Ber, Bev, Breifne, Brid, Calli, Carmel, Carol, Carole, Caroline, Carolyn, Catherine, Cathy, Clare, Claire, Christine, Christina, Chiara, Ciara, Clodagh, Collette, Cora, David, Deirdre, Denise, Diarmuid, Doreen, Dot, Eithne, Eileen, Eilis, Eimear, Elaine, Edel, Emma, Emer, Enda, Fiona, Frances, Gemma, Georgina, Ger, Gillian, Grace, Grainne, Hanna, Hannah, Hilary, Helen, Irene, Jacinta, Jenny, Jan, Jackie, James, Janice, Jessica, Joanne, Josie, Judy, Julie, Julia, Karen, Kathy, Katy, Kathryn, Kathleen, Laura, Lisa, Lissy, Lorna, Lorraine, Linda, Lynda, Lynn, Lyzelle, Louise, Lucinda, Lucy, Maeve, Mandy, Marian, Marie, Martin, Maurette, Melinda, Miriam, Margaret, Mags, Maria, Martina, Mary, Marlou, Maz, Michelle, Michael, Miriam, Nettie, Niamh, Noreen, Noirin, Norah, Norma, Orla, Pat, Paul, Paula, Pauline, Patricia, Rachel, Rose, Rosie, Ruth, Oonagh, Rita, Ria, Rob, Roberta, Roseanne, Sarah, Sandy, Sandra, Sharon, Sheena, Shona, Sinead, Siobhan, Sue, Susan, Suzie, Sylvia, Silvia, Toni, Tracey, Trish, Jennie, Una, Ursula, Val, Valerie, Vanessa, Vera, Yvonne, Zina... (I could go on).

I thank the Lukes' most cherished Liverpool friends for their enduring affection and love over three decades: Brian and Celia O'Connor, Jon and Chrissie Nelson, Nick and Carmel Manley, David and Moira Ritchie, Tony and Jane Good, Andy Jones, Paul Mullins, Kieran O'Driscoll Jr, Jill and Allan Whalley, Austin and Helen Carty, and Mick and Catherine Fitzpatrick.

I thank our neighbours and friends in Ballintemple for their occasionally life-saving, always life-enhancing, friendship,

Acknowledgements

particularly 'the two Captains' John and Liz Butler, my confidants Conan Lynch and Anne Marie Linehan, Gareth and Carole Kendellen, Joe and Liz Brosnan, Maeve and Killian Hurley, Joyce and Johnny Kerins, Billy and Rachel Stack, Terry and Jackie English, Jim and Lynn Oliver, Vinnie and Maura McDermott, Cathal and Marie McBride, Liam Tuohy and Maire Crowley, Donal and Gillian Johnston, Pearse and Ann Sreenan, John Horan, Tony and Dorothy Kehoe, Roddy Galvin, Paul Murray and Niall MacMahon, and the Van Haastrechts of Amsterdam and Ballintemple.

I also thank the squad of junior coaches at Cork Constitution FC for their comradeship over many Saturdays, and especially during the unforgettable trip to Paris in 2014, and since: Neil Collins, Frank Coombes, Malcolm Coomber, Denis Kennelly, Mick Moloney, Peter Morehead, Ray Murray, Paul O'Callaghan, Ray O'Leary, and John McHenry.

I particularly thank some former medical 'trainees' for their uninterrupted support during my most difficult times: Ashley Bhageerutty, Elspeth Worthington, Ian Norton, Jean O'Sullivan, Ger O'Connor, Hilary Fallon, Louise Kenny, Anne Weaver, Fionnghaile Nixon, Andrew Maxwell, Shane Kukaswadia, Jeff Mulcaire, Maeve Leonard, and Norman Pao. I sometimes feel that younger doctors do not fully appreciate how much older doctors like – and need – to be around them. But I have long been grateful for the company and comradeship of young enthusiastic colleagues.

I am very grateful to many medical colleagues in Cork for their simple friendliness when I *really* needed it, including: Drs Neil Brennan, Gemma Browne, Gary Lee, Sheila O'Sullivan, Colm Henry, David Curran, Brian McNamara, Brian Sweeney, Simon Cronin, Charlie Marks, Morgan

McCourt, Emmet Andrews, Peter Kearney, Eddie Fitzgerald, Micheal O'Riordain, Michael Maher, Chris Cotter, Seamus O'Mahony, George Fitzgerald, Harry Kelleher, Tom Cahill, Jeff Featherstone, Tony Lynch, Claire McCarthy, Evelyn McGrath, Joe Dillon, Mick Crotty, Eddie O'Sullivan, Barry Oliver, Pat Lee, Mehboob Kukaswadia, Paula O'Leary, Denis O'Mahony, Mick Molloy, Sinead Harney, Michael Moore, Aisling Campbell, Louise Burke, Fergus Shanahan, George Shorten, Charlie Marks, Eugene Cassidy, Neil O'Donovan, Simon Blake, Matthew Murphy, Sean T O'Sullivan, Eoin O'Broin, Orna O'Toole, Ciaran Brady, Jason Kelly, Duncan Sleeman, Pat Fleming, Cathy Dewhurst, Criostóir O Súilleabháin, Anita Griffith, Clodagh Keohane, Mark Dolan, Mary Horgan, Fergus Shanahan, and Arthur Jackson.

I offer my limitless appreciation, admiration and gratitude to all my comrades in the emergency medicine community in Cork and beyond, for their friendship (and tolerance), especially Steve Cusack, Gemma Kelleher, Gerry McCarthy, Iomhar O'Sullivan, Conor Deasy, Adrian Murphy, Jason Van Der Velde, Kanti Dasari, Rory O'Brien, Darren McLoughlin, Eoin Fogarty, Ronan O'Sullivan, Fergal Cummins, Kieran Henry, Hugh Doran and ex officio Gerry O'Dwyer. And I particularly thank Steve and Rosemary Cusack for their kindness and magnanimity over three decades to the Luke family.

For their unwavering loyalty, affection, countless good times and help when it was needed, I sincerely thank the Lukes' dearest and oldest 'new friends' in Cork: the Finns (Bairbre, John, Fiona, Kitty, Zara and Emilie), the Hayes (Ally, Ian, Edward, Hannah and Sean) the Hurleys of Castle Mary (Brid, Des, Donagh and Emmett), the Spinks of Great

Acknowledgements

Island (Jan and Alistair), the Murphys of Harty's Quay (Eoin and Cliona) and the McNultys of Ardmore (Betty and James). And, similarly, I thank my favourite Irish emergency physician, Dr Una Geary; my favourite Irish radiologist, Professor Jim Meaney; and my favourite emergency physician in Oz, Dr David Eddey, for their friendship and support over many years.

Finally, I express my immense gratitude to those medical colleagues who cared for me in recent times, and whose expertise and empathy were so crucial, therapeutic and appreciated: Dr Nuala O'Connor, Professor John Gallagher, Dr Tom Cahill, Dr Jenny Shine, Dr Ronan Margey, Dr David Curran, Mr George Kaar, Professor Anthony Clare, Professor Abbie Lane, Professor Mick Molloy, Dr Brian McNamara, Mr Colm Taylor, and – for the past 30 years – Dr Mark Phelan. This doctor-patient would simply not have been here now, looking forward to the future with optimism and enthusiasm, without their professionalism, wisdom, and compassion.

CL, June 2021